Quantum Healing with the Biofeedback L.I.F.E. System

ANDREA BERGER

ISBN: 978-1500145705

Printed in Charleston, South Carolina, USA
CreateSpace Independent Publishing Platform

To Michael

Contents

Acknowledgments

I am deeply grateful to my family for their undying support over the years: Michael Berger, Alexander Berger, Helen Berger, Natalia Turcu and Raluca Koch; to the Atlantic University faculty who advised me through my Culminating Project, the basis of this book: John Amoroso, Ph.D., Committee Chairperson and Candis Collins, M.S.W., M.A., Committee Member; to Carol Sabick de la Herran of the Monroe Institute, who encouraged my passion for energy healing; and to Linda Henderson, H.D., D.T.C.M., Department Head of Energy Medicine and Biofeedback at the College of International Holistic Studies, who trained me in the use of the L.I.F.E. System™.

Disclaimer

Biofeedback with the L.I.F.E. System™ is not a substitute for effective standard medical, dental, chiropractic or psychotherapy treatment. It assists in achieving Stress Management, Muscle Relaxation and Preventative Healthcare, and is not intended to diagnose, treat, cure or prevent any disease.

The views and opinions expressed in this book are those of the author and do not reflect the official policy or position of the L.I.F.E. System inventors, manufacturers and distributors. The L.I.F.E. System client sessions described in this book are only examples and should not be utilized in real-world health care decision making, as they are based only on limited information.

Introduction

I have always felt attracted to energy healing and energy medicine. As a teenager in Romania, I met a clairvoyant lady who was using her hands to do energy healing. She taught me how to do it and it felt natural to me, as if I was "remembering" it. Later in life, I became a Reiki Master and a Vortexhealing® advanced practitioner.

During a trip to Romania in the Spring of 2012, I met a biofeedback therapist who conducted a healing session on me and was able to identify and release an emotional trauma from when I was 13 years old.

I became intrigued about this healing modality and upon my return to the US, researched it and purchased the Living Information Forms Energy (L.I.F.E.) biofeedback system. The inventor, Chris Keser, is a veteran homeopath who has worked with energy medicine and biofeedback since the 1970's.

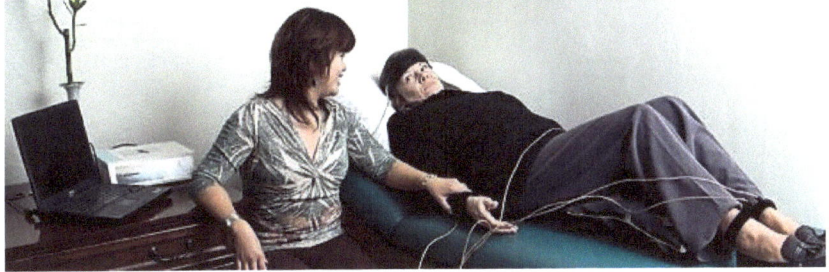

L.I.F.E. is an advanced electro-physiological biofeedback device, which, according to the manufacturer's website, has been "rigorously tested, including some double-blind studies." It is CE-certified throughout the European Union as a Class 2A medical instrument and it is also registered in the United States, Australia, and South Africa as a biofeedback device.

Training and certification as biofeedback practitioner for the L.I.F.E. System™ is provided by the College of International Holistic Studies (C.I.H.S.) in Canada. I completed the training and received my biofeedback diploma in October 2012 and later took some more advanced training. I have worked with many clients, often with amazing results. The system helps reduce stress and promotes balance of the physical, emotional, mental and spiritual energy bodies with the aid of 14,000+ frequencies, including Rife, meridians, and homeopathic frequencies. The L.I.F.E system also has the ability to identify past lives and to send balancing frequencies to the unresolved conflicts from those lives.

Quantum Physics and Quantum Healing

Quantum physics has revolutionized the way we think about our world. As our scientific knowledge grows and more sophisticated research is conducted, the theories of quantum physics are slowly being proven. While matter may appear solid to our eyes, science has determined that at a subatomic level matter is composed of tiny energy particles spinning very fast in an empty space. It appears that this spinning energy is influenced by consciousness (or observation). The famous "double-slit experiment" to determine if a photon behaves like energy (wave) or matter (particle) shows that the photon acts like a particle if the experiment is observed by a conscious observer, and like a wave if it's not observed. Quantum physicists speculate that the universe is filled with "dark energy" and "dark matter," weakly interacting with ordinary matter, causing the Universe to expand. Similarly, metaphysicists believe the universe is filled with "subtle energy" and "subtle matter," which is non-physical, hard to measure, appears to be influenced by our mind and is impacting our physical body (Henderson, 2009, p. 10).

Deepak Chopra defines quantum healing as the ability of the mind to spontaneously correct the mistakes of the body. He believes that our physical bodies are "intelligent fields of energy," containing the needed information to maintain equilibrium and health. Quantum healing involves a shift in these fields of energy, resulting in a correction of an idea that has gone wrong. In his view, quantum healing involves "healing one mode of consciousness (mind) to bring about changes in another mode of consciousness (body)" (Chopra, 1989, p. 241).

Quantum healing is still in its infancy, but quantum physics has already inspired several quantum healing devices, which act similarly to traditional biofeedback devices, only the biofeedback is based on "subtle energies" that are more difficult to quantify and measure. The connection of these devices to a client's body is through the subtle energy field and it appears that distance is not a factor. These devices measure the subtle energy pulse of the brain, the subtle energy of the muscle activity, and the subtle energy associated with heart rate variability (Henderson, 2009, p. 11).

Royal Raymond Rife, a medical doctor and inventor of the Universal Microscope in the late 1920s, was able to observe cancer viruses through his microscope, and discovered that exposing a virus to certain frequencies killed it quickly. After many years of experimentation, Rife invented the Rife Frequency Instrument, a device that produced the exact frequencies needed to destroy various disease organisms (Lynes, 2009, p. 15). In 1934, he successfully used this instrument to heal people of many illnesses, including cancer. These special "Rife frequencies" are available today in several biofeedback devices, including the L.I.F.E. system.

Quantum biofeedback devices identify stress patterns in the body on thousands of different organs, bones, muscles, hormones, emotional states, energy meridians, viruses, bacteria, food-related sensitivities, and much more. These systems not only identify the stressors, but they also send healthy energy frequencies back to the client's body to help it restore health (Cook, 2004, p. 318).

Edgar Cayce on Holistic Healing

Cayce was the forerunner in the West of the idea that one must focus on the "whole patient" in any treatment, not just a particular organ; that body, mind and spirit must be treated together, not in isolation; that the focus should be on prevention rather than on the disease; that medication is not always necessary for healing; and that self-empowerment and self-healing are important components to treatment. According to Cayce, in order to heal ourselves and grow spiritually, we must change hindering attitudes and our thinking patterns, as "mind is the builder" (Reading 1747-5). We need to overcome fear, doubt and anger, which control so many people's lives. Edgar Cayce was able to heal many people by recommending castor oil packs, tonics, herbs, and the use of electrical appliances. He also recommended prayer and meditation, in order to change negative attitudes and emotions. The key to healing, in Edgar Cayce's view, is for the body to be in harmony spiritually, mentally and physically.

My own approach to health and healing is compatible with Cayce's ideas and principles. I believe that a healthy lifestyle, diet and exercise are important to wellbeing, enabling one to reach harmony and balance between body, mind and spirit. An illness is a signal that the system is out of balance, and it is important to not just treat the symptoms, but to address the whole system. Thus, healing is multi-dimensional and in order to achieve and maintain health, all three dimensions, body, mind and spirit, need to be addressed, as they are interconnected.

There are several aspects of healing and wellbeing, such as the quality of life and empowerment of the person seeking improved health. Having a strong desire to be healed, a good diet, exercise, relaxation, and having loving relationships are helpful factors in promoting good health. To maintain wellbeing, it is also important that people have a life purpose, and focus on the present, rather than live in the past or future.

Edgar Cayce recommended in many readings the use of a few unusual appliances and devices which use electrical energy for healing (Reading 3491-1). Some of these appliances make use of the electromagnetic spectrum (e.g., Violet Ray Appliance and Ultra Violet Ray Light Therapy) and others were said to be using "vibrational energy" of a low electrical nature (e.g., the Radium or Radial Appliance, and the Wet Cell Battery). The low electrical energy was described by Cayce as being the life force, or creative force, within the body (Reading 3491-1). This is similar to the "subtle energy" mentioned nowadays in quantum healing. Cayce's "vibrational energy" devices seem to work on a similar principle as the quantum biofeedback devices of today, balancing the body's natural energies.

The L.I.F.E. Biofeedback System

The L.I.F.E. System uses biofeedback and bioresonance to energetically stimulate the body's own healing mechanisms. It scans and harmonizes the body's stresses and imbalances energetically, in a non-invasive way. By sending balancing frequencies to the body, it reduces the disease-inducing stressors, thus helping the body return to its natural state of health. It facilitates self-awareness and self-responsibility that fosters balance of the mind-body system.

The L.I.F.E. System is one of the most modern and innovative biofeedback devices on the market today. It is safe, powerful, and user-friendly, relying on 20+ years of research conducted in the field of bio-energetic and bio-response medicine. The system measures the reaction to many individual vibrational signals using voltage, amperage, and resistance. While some biofeedback systems offer one-way therapy, the L.I.F.E. System sends and receives signals. It also evaluates and changes the signal/therapy, depending on the client's needs.

A few years ago, the inventor, Chris Keser, described the L.I.F.E. system as follows at a seminar in Nice, France:

"This system took nearly four years to develop, and I'm pleased with the result. We will continue to develop the system and add other functions. This for me is much more than just the development of a biofeedback program – it has been a labor of love more than anything else. I truly believe the future of medicine lies in the understanding of energy fields and our ability to make changes within the energy fields. I believe that all disease has an energy component / emotional level disturbance lying behind it, resulting in an imbalance in the energy field. ... This is the future of the 21st century."

The human body has electromagnetic vibrational patterns that have resonance, reactance, and self-correcting capacities. Each cell in the body, each organ, operates at a certain vibrational frequency, and combined, they form a vibrational energy pattern unique to each individual, a distinctive "thumbprint," or "address" in the universe. Every human thought, emotion, and action has a certain vibrational frequency. Viruses, bacteria, fungi, parasites, diseases, etc. also have resonant energy patterns. These energy vibrations can be measured with the L.I.F.E System as voltage, amperage and resistance (Henderson, 2010, p. 6).

The physical body's primary electrical systems, which can be measured by the L.I.F.E. system, are: 1) the Nervous System (the brain, neurons, and nerves which cause muscle contractions, nerve transmission, glandular secretion, and sensation); and 2) the Electromagnetic System (energy emanating from atoms and cells; these vibrations have been called an "aura" or a person's "energy field").

Our cells keep our bodies in harmony. Feelings, thoughts and the emotions we experience impact the cells in our body either negatively or positively. Lifestyles can also create damaging energy patterns, which are stored in cells and may build up unnoticed for years (Henderson, 2010, p. 7).

Stress induces an alarm response in the body, which will provoke symptoms. Stress can come from many sources such as emotional issues, toxicity, trauma, deficiency, perverse energy, pathogens, allergy, habits, heredity and mental factors. If the stress continues, the body will go into an adaptation stage, which could be symptom free. A lack of symptoms is not necessarily a sign of good health. The client can have a life-threatening disease and be symptom free, as a disease can be present in the body years before any medical device can detect it (e.g. breast cancer is present in the body long before it registers on a mammogram). As the stress continues, the disease, unless it is treated, progresses.

Many therapies/medications just suppress the symptoms, interrupting the body's signal that there is a serious imbalance. Rather than eliminating the symptoms, an effective therapy helps the body selfregulate, restoring balance and proper function.

The L.I.F.E. System can detect energetic aberrations (a state or condition markedly different from the norm) and repair them. The L.I.F.E. System is exchanging information with the client's body using harnesses attached to the forehead, ankles and wrists. These harnesses are made of special conductive silicone, which allows for very low-current electrical communication through the computer's USB port and a multi-functional interface box.

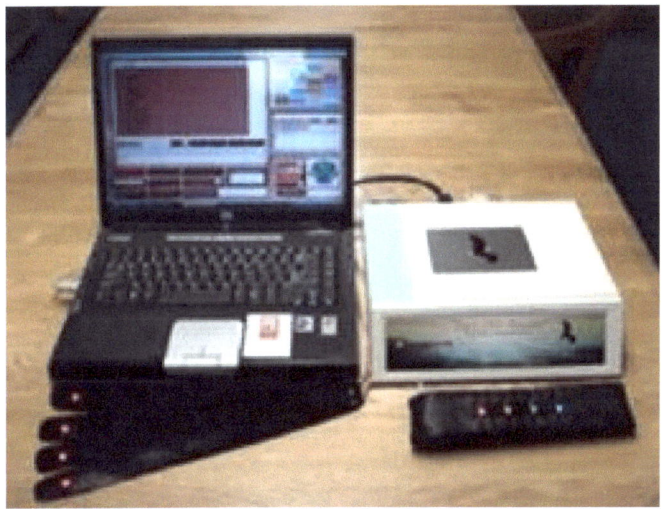

For more technical information about how the L.I.F.E. biofeedback system works, please see Appendix A.

During the testing/assessment phase, a client's biofeedback response is measured in response to nearly 7,000 individual frequency signals in 39 separate categories (e.g. allergens, bacteria, parasites, etc.). This process, called the **Reactivity Test**, takes approximately 4 to 7 minutes, depending upon the speed of the computer. The computer calculates an average value of response between 0 and 2000, which results in a list defining the client's reactions or stress potentials, indicating an exposure, weakness, predisposition or susceptibility to a specific frequency signal. The greatest energy disturbances will be recorded and displayed at the top of the list (see screen print below). Each item has its own distinctive, complex waveform, which is graphically viewed and represented by a unique fractal image. Additionally, the Reactivity Test panel contains a detailed description of each item.

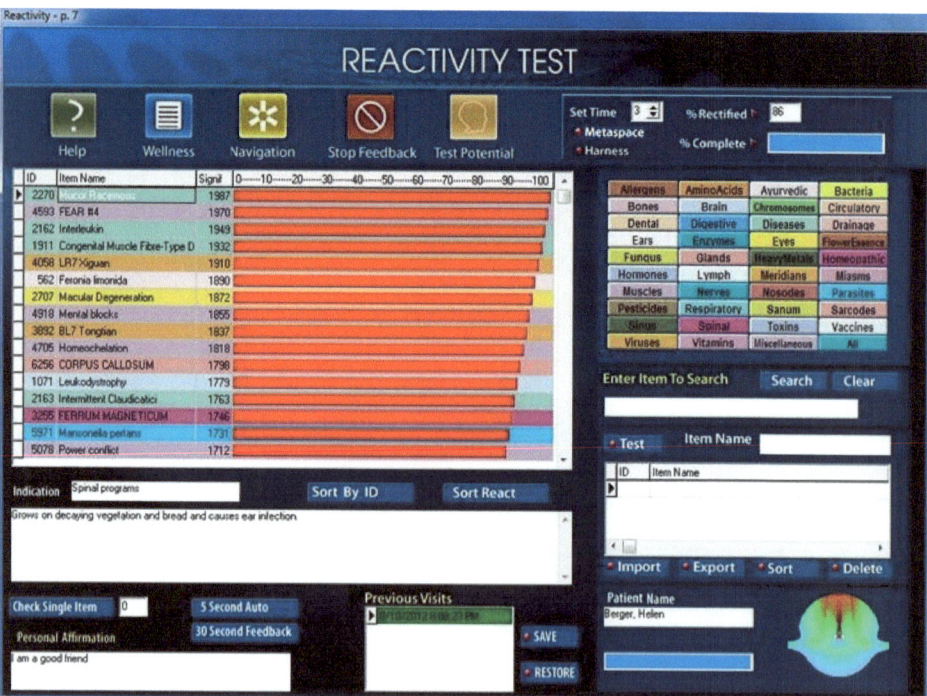

Once the Reactivity Test is complete, the system recommends a therapy course in the "Indication" field, e.g. Cell-Com, Chakra/Color, Rife-Like, Meridian, Spinal, or Neuro-Emotional Profile. The practitioner can access these programs from the **Wellness Information** panel.

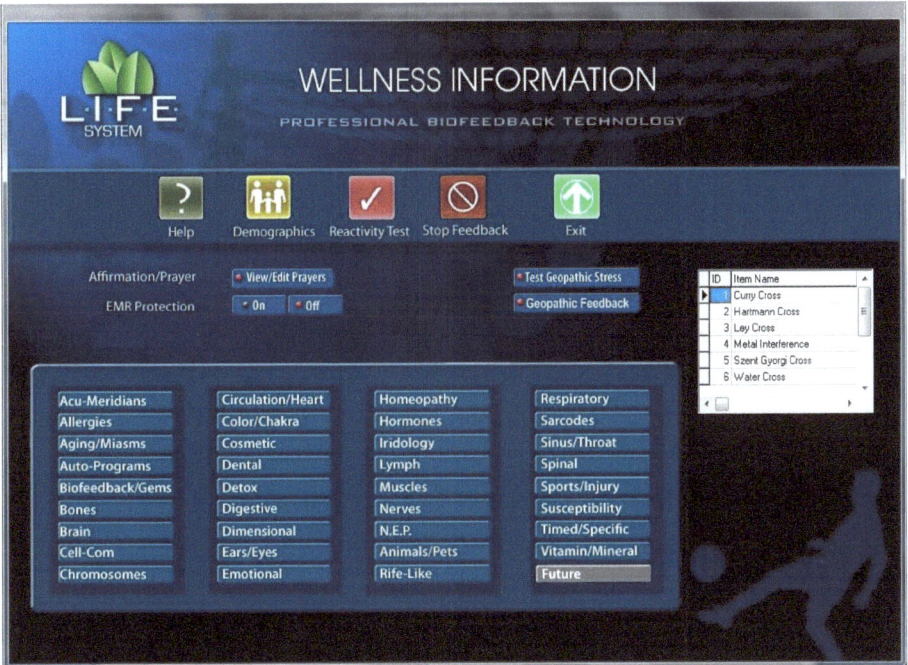

On the Wellness Information panel, the practitioner can test for **Geopathic Stress** affecting the client and then release it. This is important to do at the beginning of each session, as it facilitates the highest level of energetic balancing for the client. The next step is to go to the **Susceptibility Index** program and run an additional test in order to determine more detailed stress potentials.

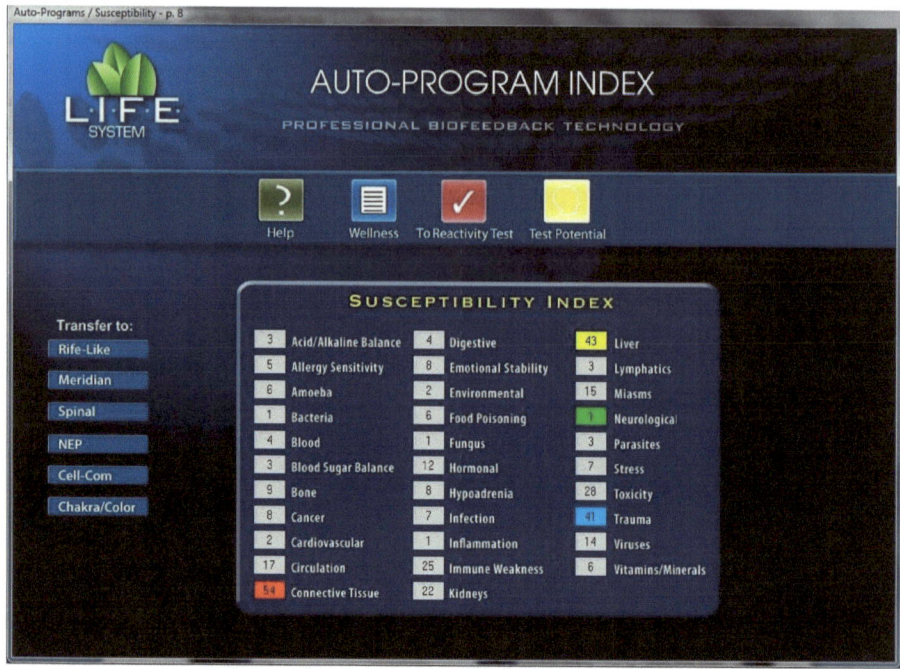

The practitioner looks at the four suggestions highlighted in red, yellow, blue and green, for further indication of what to work on during the course of the session. Given that a client session is only one hour long, the practitioner must decide wisely which of the possible programs available in the L.I.F.E. system to work with. Usually, during one session there is time for only 3 or 4 programs: the **Susceptibility Index**; the program recommended by the **Reactivity Test** (in the above Reactivity Test screen print the indicated program is the **Spinal Profile**); and one or two additional programs, selected based on the Susceptibility Index results.

My L.I.F.E. System Healing Practice

After completing my training with the College for International Holistic Studies, I started to practice on friends and family members. Some people could sense the energy moving through their body and felt much more relaxed after the session. Others had powerful emotional releases, or noticeable improvements in their physical ailments. Some people come once, out of curiosity, to have their aura measured or to find out about a past life. Others become regular clients and usually, it is these people who see the most drastic results in their health and wellbeing. As for myself, I was pleasantly surprised that my sinus problems, allergies and migraines gradually faded away, and I now rarely need any medication.

Below is a picture of my L.I.F.E. System setup:

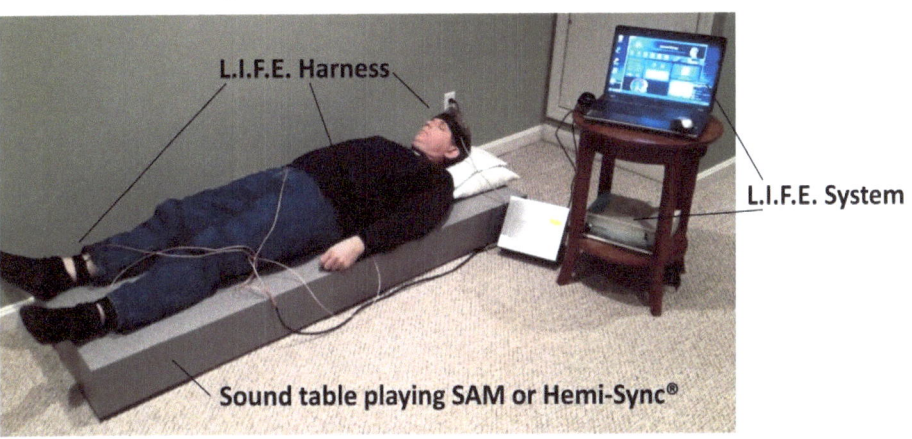

My clients have the option to lie down on a sound table and listen to relaxing, consciousness-expanding music with Hemi-

Sync® or Spatial Angle Modulation™ (SAM) audio technology from the Monroe Institute.

I have worked with 55 clients as of July 2014. Each new client signs a consent form, stating that biofeedback therapy in no way replaces conventional medical treatment. I keep detailed notes about each client session, for future reference.

Healing Sessions

Client #1

This client is a 52-year old woman suffering for a long time from stomach issues (bile duct problems) and migraines. She was also under intense stress, caused primarily by her ailing mother, and mentioned that she is not sleeping well. Below is the description of the three sessions conducted with this client.

Session One

During the first session, the L.I.F.E. Reactivity Test indicated that the client may have some thyroid imbalance, which may contribute to her migraines and stomach issues. In our conversation, the client indicated that she takes Imitrex and Maxalt for migraines and these drugs have the side effect of upset stomach, especially in women. The client also noted that she is highly sensitive to drugs and toxins.

The system-recommended program was the **Cell-Com Programs** (see screen prints in Appendix C) and the identified

Susceptibilities were Amoeba, Miasm, Acid/Alkaline, and Trauma. I made note of these items, then proceeded to the **Color/Chakra** panel. Below is her aura from the first session, prior to any energy balancing.

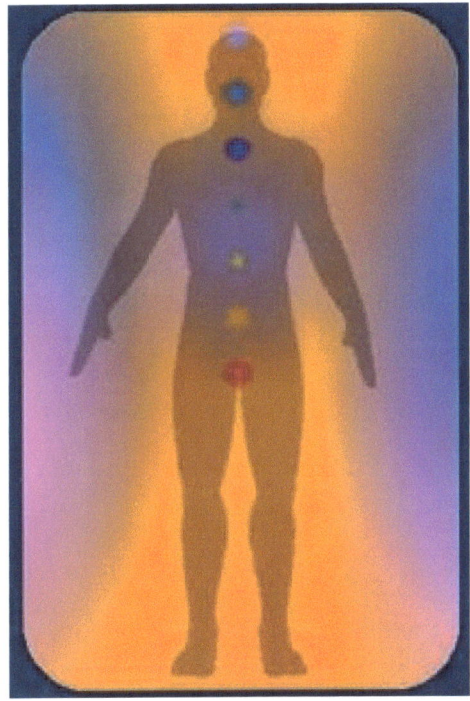

The reason I went to the Color/ Chakra panel is two-fold: 1) to enhance the client's ability to balance, having all chakras more open, with more energy flowing, and 2) I wanted a graphic representation of the client's energy field, prior to any balancing, so I can compare it to her aura after the third session.

The chakra test indicated stress in the Heart, Crown, Brow and Stomach chakras, and they all balanced except the Heart. I made a note to return to this panel in a future session.

I then proceeded to the recommended **Cell-Com Program**, where the main stressors were: "Allergy Treatment – auricular points," "Cervical Vertebral disorders," "Coxarthrosis" and "Skin Disorders & Lymphatic" problems. This was no surprise to the client, as she has degenerative disc disease and allergies. I sent balancing frequencies to these four items.

Next, I proceeded to the **Neuro-Emotional Profile**, as I felt the emotional traumas and the stress/anxiety, if balanced, may alleviate the migraines and stomach issues. Anxiety, Lust, Anger and Jealousy emerged as the main emotional stressors. Lust and Jealousy didn't balance completely, so I made a note to address these during the next session. The client's **Unconscious Self-Evaluation Hint** pointed to "Feelings of Prejudice" and balanced within 2 minutes. The client did not immediately resonate with this hint, but seemed to accept the other stressors, and we decided to embark on the **Emotional panel** in the next session, to see how this unconscious hint may relate to her other emotional stressors. Overall, the client was pleased with this session, as she felt that the system had pinpointed stress areas that were significant to her.

Session Two

The client reported having been sick during the week with stomach flu. Given the changing weather, the migraines did not let down either. She continued to stay up late and thus got only a few hours of sleep per night, but she got some better rest during the weekend. On the emotional front, however, the client felt that she had made some progress, feeling less stressed and anxious in her interactions with her mother.

Her **Susceptibilities** were Blood, Viruses, Allergy Sensitivity and Lymphatics, which seemed somewhat consistent with the stressors from the last session (allergies, lymph). After sending balancing energy to all items which didn't fully balance during the last session, I then went to the **Rife-Like Organ Profile**. Here the main stressors were Heart, Cervical, Stomach and Sexual Organs. It is interesting that Cervical and Sexual Organs came out, as the client had reported benign cysts in her ovaries, breasts, and other areas of the body, that she has had on and off for many years. Stomach again showed up as a stress area, and it was the only one which didn't rectify above 85%, so I made a note to return to this item in the next session.

I then proceeded to the **Emotional Transformation & Timeline** Program. The client's body chose Carelessness (emotional stress), Performance Conflict (conflict stress), Healer Figure (relationship stress) and 19 years (age stress).

All these items balanced nicely, except for Healer Figure, so I made a note to address this next time. I also recorded the secondary stress factors, for future sessions. I then sent energy to the following items: Inner Peace, Stress Reduction, Well-Being, Anxiety Reduction, Ascendance and Transcendence. The reason I selected Ascendance and Transcendence is that the more in tune a person is with her Higher Self, the better equipped she is to deal with emotional and physical issues. The other reason for selecting Ascendance and Transcendence is because "Inner Guidance" showed up in the Reactivity Matrix as a significant stress factor.

Lastly, I proceeded to the **Dimensional Transformation** Program, because during calibration, the "spiritual line" connected

17

last. Also, in the Reactivity Matrix, "Inner Guidance" came up at the bottom of the list with a significance of 99%. I also know that the client is interested in the spiritual aspects of her life and practices meditation regularly. The **Transcendence Program** rebalanced at 98%. The **Past Life Portal** indicated a past life as a female shipbuilder in 1028 AD, in Europe. The conflict in that life was "Disappointment," which resonated with the client, as she has had her fair share of disappointments in her current life. This conflict rebalanced to 89% in two tries.

During the debrief at the end, the client mentioned that she had felt a lot of energy movement in her heart. As we reviewed the results from the **Emotional Transformation & Timeline** panel, she recalled her life at age 19. She was in college and described herself as a perfectionist. She became very stressed and suffered from anorexia and depression. She went to see a psychologist, who had a colleague doctor prescribe drugs for her, though this doctor never saw her in person. The drugs he prescribed caused severe allergic reactions, to the point that she developed tardive dyskinesia syndrome and eventually went into a coma, at which point the doctors finally took her off these antipsychotic drugs. We were both amazed that the L.I.F.E. system brought this up, as she had not thought about this phase in her life in a long time. Everything seemed to fit with what was going on in her life at age 19: her perfectionism (performance conflict), her conflict with her doctors (healer figure), their carelessness. In addition, she married a doctor (another "healer

18

figure"), from whom she is now divorced. The Unconscious Hint from the last session, "Feelings of Prejudice," made more sense now. It could be interpreted two-fold: 1) the doctors' prejudice against a young woman with anorexia, and/or 2) the client's (well-justified) prejudice against "healer figures."

Given the client's high interest in the L.I.F.E. system (she has an MA in Industrial Psychology), I showed her the system a bit. We went to the **Brain** panel and tested her brain balance, then applied feedback. At this point, she was not connected to the harness anymore, so the feedback was applied in "virtual mode." We also looked at the **Biofeedback** panel and tested her gem preference, which was Amazonite, Dioptase and Pyrite. I applied feedback for a couple of minutes. We then concluded the session, which we both found to be very informative and productive.

Session Three

The client reported that her benign cysts were acting up again (she's had this condition for years) and that she went to the doctor to remove some of her ovarian fibroid cysts. Her migraines were still there, but were perhaps somewhat better, as she was taking less medication. Her sleep had improved slightly, as did her stress level. She continued to see progress on the emotional front as well.

Her **Susceptibilities** this time around were Hypoadrenia, Neurological, Parasites and Environmental. I made a note of these stressors and planned to address them in future sessions.

Hypoadrenia seems very relevant to the client's condition, as it signifies reduced function of the adrenal glands. The adrenal glands sit on top of the kidneys and help the body deal with stress, including emotional and environmental stress. Fatigue is one of the symptoms of Hypoadrenia, and so is weight gain and depression. Adrenal stress can also be caused by parasites, viruses and allergies.

After sending balancing energy to all items which didn't fully balance during the last session, I went to the **Neuro-Emotional Profile** and sent frequencies to Depression, which balanced to 81%. I then tested the client's **Unconscious Self-Evaluation Hint**, and to my surprise, the same one as in the first session came up: "Feelings of Prejudice." It balanced in two tries to 91%.

Next, I proceeded to the **Emotional Transformation & Timeline** program to work on the stressors that were identified during the last session. These were "Constant brooding over trauma" (emotional stress), Sleep Conflict (conflict stress), Idol Figure (relationship stress) and 35 years (age stress). I chose to rebalance "Mother" instead of "Idol Figure," given her intense emotional relationship with her mother. All items rebalanced nicely, so I made a note to address the Idol Figure next time. I also sent frequencies to "Healer Figure," to "Anxiety" and "Stress Reduction," given that they didn't fully balance last time.

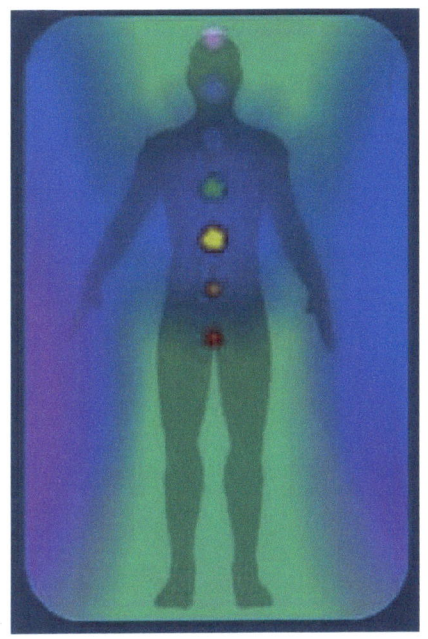

Lastly, I went to the **Color Chakra Profile**, to take a snapshot of her aura. After the session, when I showed this picture to the client, she resonated very much with these colors, as green and blue are her favorite colors and she attributed the green color to her emerging healing. The description of the colors in the system also seemed to fit her personality and current emotional state.

During the debrief, we discussed the items from the **Emotional Transformation & Timeline** panel. It turns out that at age 35, the client moved into a new house in another neighborhood. It was then when she started having night terrors and vivid dreams, which eventually allowed her to recall a trauma she had when she was 7 years old. She remembered that in this very neighborhood, her mother tried to kill her when she was 7 years old, by abandoning her in the car in the middle of a street, just past the top of a hill, so that incoming cars couldn't see the car as they were coming up the hill. Her mother (who was battling depression, mental issues and alcoholism at the time) got out of the

21

car, ordered her to go in the back seat (unbuckled), and watched from the side-line as a car came up the hill and hit their car from behind, causing the 7-year old girl to be catapulted into the windshield. She was rushed to the hospital, where she was treated for head injuries. Since that "accident," her personality changed and she started having sleep issues and bouts of depression. We were both amazed that the system had picked up on this trauma. This incident explains the "constant brooding over trauma" (which she has carried with her since she was 7 years old), the sleep conflict, the "Idol Figure" (her mother) and the fact that she recollected this suppressed, long-ago trauma at age 35, when she moved into the neighborhood where the trauma occurred. Her head injury at age 7 might also explain the migraines she has suffered from all her life, and the "brain" stressors the system uncovered in the reactivity matrix (cerebral cortex, frontal lobe, TMJ). The unconscious hint "Feelings of Prejudice" also makes sense in this context.

The client is very interested in continuing with these sessions. In future sessions, I plan to continue to work on the Emotional Program, as this one seemed to have "struck gold" twice so far, uncovering deep, unresolved traumas. I plan to also address the Hormones, Aging/Miasms, Allergies, Digestive Programs, and the Rife-Like Program, to strengthen her system with the goal towards detoxification.

Client #2

This client is a 57-year old woman, who came to me complaining about chronic pain, especially in her upper back, and arthritis. She told me she had a plethora of other health issues, such as bursitis (knee), gout, ulcers, bladder issues, hypertension, allergies and attention deficit disorder (ADD). She was also interested in dealing with her addictions to tobacco and food. Over a period of eight months, I have seen this client 5 times. Below are three of the most relevant sessions.

Session One

During our first session, the L.I.F.E. system identified the following susceptibility areas: Neurological, Hormonal, Hypoadrenia and Cardiovascular. The **Reactivity Test** recommended working with the **Color Chakra Profile**, where further tests indicated imbalances of the Base (1st chakra), Brow (6th chakra), Crown (7th chakra) and Stomach (3rd chakra), which I proceeded to balance. The color with which the client resonated most at that time was purple, so I sent frequencies of this color to her. Her aura was violet, lavender and blue, colors the client very much resonated with, and which signify intuition, imagination and peacefulness.

Given that one of the client's susceptibility areas was "Hypoadrenia," I went to the **Organ Specific Sarcodes** panel and sent balancing frequencies to the Adrenals.

Also, because one of the client's susceptibility areas was "Neurological," I went to the **Neuro-Emotional Profile**, where a further test indicated the following stress factors: Joy (or lack thereof), Depression, Carelessness and Hesitation. The "Unconscious Self Evaluation Hint" test revealed "Too Much Self Focus." I proceeded to send balancing frequencies to all of these items.

Lastly, I proceeded to the **Emotional Transformation & Timeline Profile** and sent the following frequencies: Inner Peace, Addiction Reduction, Well Being and Nicotine Withdrawal. A further test on this panel revealed the following stress factors: Friendship (emotional stress), Reliability (conflict stress), Sex Figure (relationship stress), and 12-years old (age timeline). I proceeded to send balancing frequencies to all these items. When discussing this with the client at the end of the session, she didn't know what to make of it, but the next time I saw her, she told me that she had discussed this with her sister, who remembered a male family friend from their childhood, who had molested them around the time the client was 12-years old. The client was amazed that this repressed traumatic event was picked up by the L.I.F.E. system and was brought to the surface for processing and healing.

Session Two

During this session we discussed the sexual trauma identified in the previous session. The client also reported some psychic events (e.g., communicating with a ghost) and she expressed interest in the spiritual/dimensional aspects of the L.I.F.E. system. Physically, her knee was better, she was fighting a cold and she had passed a stone. Overall, she felt that the system was helping her. The **Susceptibilities** test revealed the following imbalances: Neurological, Emotional, Inflammation and Hypoadrenia. Given that "Hypoadrenia" was once again listed as imbalance, I went to the **Organ Specific Sarcodes** panel and sent balancing frequencies to the Adrenals. Also, to Kidneys and Circulation (which appeared as susceptibility areas in the first session). I then went to the **Timed/Specific Panel**, where I applied frequencies to Arthritis, Fibromyalgia, Backache, Bladder, Bursitis, Gout and Hypertension. These were all issues that the client had complained about. Then, on the **Digestive Profile**, I sent frequencies to "Ulcers," as this was another problem the client complained about. On the **Hormone Profile**, I did a "3 minute ovarian stimulation." On the **Brain Profile**, I did an ADD and ADHD test, then sent frequencies to both these areas. I also sent frequencies for "Left Brain-Right Brain-Harmonic Balance."

I then went to the **Emotional Transformation** panel and sent frequencies to the following items: Behavior Change,

Nicotine Withdrawal, Addiction Reduction, Past Life Regression and Inner Peace.

Lastly, I went to the **Dimensional Transformation** Panel, given the client's interest in the spiritual/dimensional aspect of the L.I.F.E. system. I then used the "Past Life Portal" to reveal a past life as a male herdsman/shepherd in North America in 290 A.D. The unresolved conflict from that life was "Despair," so I sent frequencies to balance that conflict. After the session, the client really resonated with this past life. She actually remembered a past life as a Native American boy, who lost his best friend due to some accident and felt despair and guilt his entire life. The client was amazed that the L.I.F.E. system picked up on this past life and conflict and she felt much more at peace at the end of the session.

Session Three

The client reported feeling better physically. She had less pain and had been placed on reduced medication by her doctor. However, she was now on steroids for her Achilles tendon injury. Emotionally, she reported feeling better.

The system identified the following susceptibility areas: Bacteria, Allergy, Hormonal and Toxicity. The **Reactivity Test** recommended working with the **Neuro-Emotional Profile**, where further tests indicated the following imbalances: Jealousy, Impulsivity, Confusion and Delusion. The "Unconscious Self Evaluation Hint" test revealed "Explore Family Conflict." I proceeded to send balancing frequencies to all these items. When discussing this with the client at the end of the session, she told me that this makes sense, as she was in the process of taking custody over her granddaughter, due to her daughter-in-law's inability to care for the child.

During the third session, I also went to the **Lymph Profile**, where I sent frequencies to Lymph Plaque and Lymph Stasis, as well as a 2-minute special stimulation. Strengthening her lymphatic system will help her reduce toxicity in her body. From the **Respiratory Profile**, I sent her frequencies for balancing Bronchitis and Chronic Cough. From the **Muscles, Cartilage & Ligaments** panel I sent her frequencies for Bursitis, Achilles Tendon, Tendonitis and Gout. I then went to the **Organ Specific Sarcodes** panel to send frequencies for Adrenals, Thyroid and Bladder. I then went to the **Detox & Multiple Stress Profile** to send frequencies for Full Body Detox and Bacteria, given that her susceptibilities were Bacteria and Toxicity. Lastly, I sent the following frequencies from the **Emotional Transformation** panel: Nicotine Withdrawal, Addiction Reduction and Conflict Resolution.

Overall, I am pleased with the progress this client has made over the course of the L.I.F.E. sessions. She has since attended several meditation workshops to further her spiritual and emotional transformation. She is better able to handle her health issues, which she claims have improved.

Client #3

This client is a 61-year old woman who came to me complaining about her chronic cough, depression, and toxicity. In our first session the client confessed that she had been molested as a child and wanted, if possible, to heal that aspect of her life. The client also mentioned that she was under intense stress, caused by her ailing husband, who is suffering from terminal cancer. Over a period of five months, I have seen this client 11 times. In this paper, I will describe three of the most relevant sessions.

Session One

During our first session, the L.I.F.E. system identified the following susceptibility areas: Toxicity, Bone, Immune Weakness, and Acid/Alkaline Balance. The system also recommended working with the **Chromosome & Gene Profile**. Further tests on this panel identified the following items that needed energy balancing: "Zinc, normalization of," "Emotional blocks," "Mammary Glands," and "Fever, increased pulse and breathing."

I proceeded to balance these items, sending up to 3 minutes of balancing frequencies to each of these stressors. I also sent balancing frequencies to "All Genes" and "All Chromosomes," as well as to "Acid/Alkaline Balance," as this was identified earlier as a stress factor.

Given the client's chief complaint of chronic cough, I then proceeded to the **Respiratory Profile** and sent balancing frequencies to "Asthma" and "Bronchitis," as well as the "2 minute Special Stimulation." Then I went to the **Lymph Profile** and sent "2 minute Special Stimulation" balancing frequencies. This was followed by the **Organ Specific Sarcodes Profile**, where I sent balancing frequencies to "Bone," "Immune System" and "Metabolic."

On the **Detox & Multiple Stress Profile**, I conducted a test of the "Personal & Self Induced Stress Factors," which indicated the following items: Pork/Beef Toxins, Mental Toxins, Intestinal Toxins, and Alcohol. I then proceeded to balance these items. At the end of the session, the client confirmed that she had sensitivities to all of these items.

Lastly, I went to the **Neuro-Emotional Profile**, where a further test indicated the following stress factors: Recklessness, Projection, Fear and Impulsivity. The "Unconscious Self Evaluation Hint" test revealed "Explore Fear of Rejection." I proceeded to send balancing frequencies to all of these items. During our discussion at the end of the session, the client resonated with all of these items. Overall, the client found the session very relaxing and she could sense the energy moving through her body. She also felt that her chronic cough had eased up a bit during the session.

Session Two

The client reported less coughing at the start of the session, so we decided to focus on Emotional stressors and Detox during this session. She was particularly interested in Detox, as a medical intuitive had recently told her that she had metal and other toxicity in her body. Toxicity had also been identified by the L.I.F.E. system during the first session. The **Susceptibility Panel** indicated Environmental, Digestive, Liver, Food Poisoning and Bacteria as main stressors, so I proceeded to the **Organ Specific Sarcodes** Panel, where I sent frequencies to the Adrenals, Lungs, Digestive system, Liver, Immune system and Metabolic system.

I then proceeded to the **Circulatory Profile**, where I sent "2 minute Special Stimulation" and "Chelation Stimulation" frequencies to the circulatory system. On the **Respiratory Profile**, I sent balancing energy to Asthma and Bronchitis, as well as the overall "2 minute Special Stimulation" to the entire system. I then went to the **Detox Profile**, where I was able to balance Bacteria, Sugar Toxins and Food Toxins. I also completed the "5 minute Auto-Feedback" for overall detoxification and balancing. Lastly, I proceeded to the **Emotional Transformation Panel**, which revealed the following stress factors: Listless (emotional stress), Cultural Conflict (conflict stress), Daughter (relationship stress), and 59-years old (age timeline). I proceeded to send balancing frequencies to all these items. When discussing this with the client at the end of the session, it turns out that she indeed had a stressful event when she was 59 years old. Her daughter was moving to Chicago and this caused her to be depressed and listless.

Session Three

The client reported less stress and somewhat less coughing at the start of the session. It was time for another "Reactivity Matrix" test, which recommended the **Meridian Profile**. The **Susceptibility Panel** indicated Allergy Sensitivity, Circulation, Kidneys and Parasites. I proceeded to the **Meridian Profile**, where a further test indicated imbalances in the Governing Vessel, Bladder, Conception Vessel and Liver Meridians. I proceeded to send balancing frequencies to these meridians. Another test revealed imbalances of the following acu-meridian points: PC09 (pericardium), GV27 (governing vessel), BL17 (bladder) and LI17 (liver), which I then proceeded to rebalance. I then sent frequencies to Chronic Cough from the **Sinus & Throat Profile**, to the Kidneys from the **Organ Specific Sarcodes** Panel. Then I proceeded to the **Circulatory Profile,** where I administered a "2 minute Special Stimulation" and a "Chelation stimulation." I did this because Kidneys and Circulation showed up in the **Susceptibility Panel**.

I then went to the **Allergy Profile**, where a further test identified Parsley, Rice, Household Insect Mix, and Olfactory Sensitivity as stressors. I sent balancing frequencies to all these items, then proceeded to the **Detox Profile** to balance Parasites, as this also came up in the Susceptibility Panel.

Lastly, I proceeded to the **Dimensional Transformation Panel's Past Life Portal**. The test identified a past life as a male hunter in Europe in 583 A.D. The unresolved conflict from that life was "selfishness." I proceeded to send balancing frequencies to this conflict and, at the same time, I used the integrated imagery techniques I learned at Atlantic University (Amoroso, 2012) to regress the client into that past life. Thus, the client was able to find out more details about that life and consciously participate in releasing the conflict. She recalled being a teenage boy named Alan in Poland, who liked to hunt, but his family wanted him to be a farmer. One day, instead of working the land near home, he went into the woods and upon his return he discovered that his house had been burned down and his entire family murdered by some thieves. He felt that his selfishness had caused the deaths of his family and he never forgave himself. I guided her to release this conflict by re-scripting the story and finish any unfinished business by "talking" to his family and the thieves. She was able to successfully do this and felt much lighter and more at peace afterwards. I concluded the session by sending her "Inner Peace" and "Transcendence" frequencies.

This client truly feels that the L.I.F.E. sessions are helping her relax and heal and she has been coming regularly for the last five months, as she is going through a stressful period in her life with her husband's terminal cancer and dealing with her aging mother. She has also made other positive changes in her life, such as eating a balanced diet and exercising. I am very pleased with the progress of this client, though a bit disappointed that her chronic cough, though improved, is still lingering.

Healing Past Lives

Of special interest to me is the L.I.F.E. system's **Dimensional Transformation Panel,** which includes the **Past Life Portal**.

With the help of the L.I.F.E. system, I retrieved several of my own past lives, and was able to send healing frequencies to the unresolved conflicts from those lives.

Year	Gender	Occupation	Continent	Conflict
156	Female	Clothier, Fabric Maker	Asia	Argumentative
515	Female	Trader	Australia	Fear
604	Male	Seaman	Europe	Latent Grief
674	Male	Prisoner	Europe	Indifference
1015	Female	Peasant, Beggar	Asia	Timidity
1136	Male	Healer, Physician	Asia	Indifference
1645	Female	Servant	Europe	Inability to Love
1680	Female	Trader	S. America	Inability to Love
1755	Male	Prisoner	N. America	Sadness
1776	Male	Hunter	Africa	Worry
1822	Male	Trader	S. America	Family Conflict

Note: the year depicts the time when the unresolved conflict arose in a particular life, versus the year of birth or death.

During each session, I could clearly sense the balancing frequencies, as they released the unresolved conflict from a particular past life. Some past lives triggered memories, and using the regression techniques learned at the Monroe Institute and at Atlantic University, I was able to retrieve more details from a

particular life, while concomitantly the L.I.F.E. system was
sending me balancing frequencies.

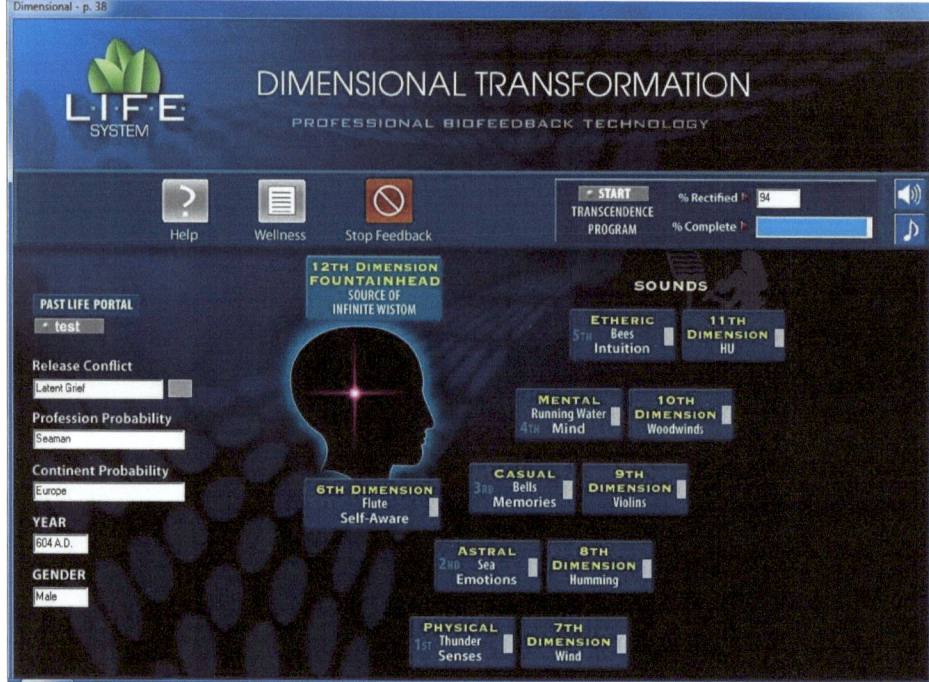

Below is my self-conducted past life regression to a life in
year 604 A.D., when I was a seaman in Europe, whose unresolved
conflict was "latent grief."

*"I am floating through space watching the Earth rotating
majestically in front of me. I focus my attention on Europe,
year 604 A.D. As I get closer, I feel a strong pull towards
Norway and decide to explore that area in more detail. I find
myself by the sea, in a small fishing community. I am a young
boy, living with my parents in a small hut. My father teaches
me how to fish and handle a fishing boat. In our village, men
make their living by fishing. In the summer, they are gone for*

*days, but when they return, we all have good food for a long
time.*

*I move now to the next important event in this life: I am a
young man with a wife and two children. I feel healthy and
happy, and life is good. I enjoy my work, fishing with my
friends and being at sea.*

*Next important event: I am stunned by grief! My family
and most our villagers are dead!! Viciously murdered during
the night by our enemies, a gang of nomad thugs on horse-
back, who came to steal from us and rape our women, then
killed them all, including our children and elders.*

*Next important event: Life has no meaning for me
anymore. I take my boat to sea and never return."*

While receiving balancing energy from the L.I.F.E. system,
I reflect on this past life and realize how my unresolved grief from
this life triggered some negative complexes, such as "inability to
love" and "indifference" in some of my future lives. I allow
myself to heal emotionally, fully and completely, as I connect
energetically with my wife and children from that life, and
recognize that they have been with me in many other lives. There
is no need to grieve for them anymore, as we are never apart.

I start to reflect on my other lives and the lessons they
provided. For example, in my lives as a trader I developed some
useful skills, such as math, business and working well with people.
My lives as a prisoner enabled me to develop a strong appreciation

for freedom, which in this life, gave me the courage to escape communist Romania and immigrate to the United States in my youth. And my life as a healer/physician in Asia may have fostered my interest in healing, yoga and meditation in this lifetime.

As a result of my L.I.F.E. sessions, I feel much more balanced and grounded emotionally. Here is a picture of my aura, captured a few months into my work with the L.I.F.E. system, including the aura color descriptions provided by the system:

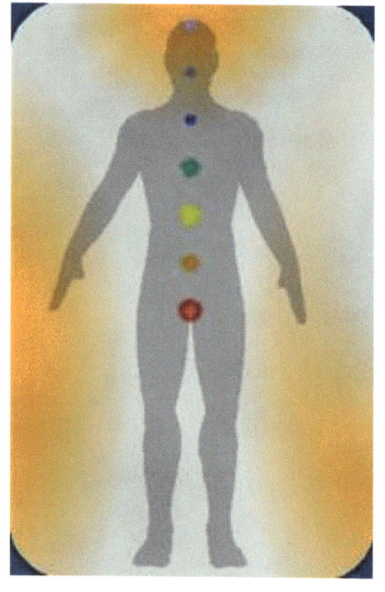

White: Transcendent, spiritual, internal thoughts and feelings, transformation, quiet, sensitive, higher dimensions, introspective.
Yellow: Playful, sunny, creative, fun, learning, light, movement, entertainer, optimism, warmth, charming, easy going.
Orange: Pleasure, enjoyment, challenge, positive, excitement, productive, physical and creative expression, adventurer, business.

I use the system regularly, especially when I work with groups of people, to keep me energized, centered and loving. During my meditation workshops, I often send L.I.F.E. spiritual frequencies to myself (e.g., Unity with All, Ascendance, Transcendence, ESP Stimulation, Astral Projection Stimulation,

Inner Awareness, Mystical Stimulation, Clairvoyance, or Inner Peace), and I find the group energy stronger and more coherent.

Input from Clients

For my Culminating Project at Atlantic University, I conducted a small research project. I sent out a questionnaire to 23 of my clients, out of which 17 responded, for a response rate of 74%. Some clients had only one L.I.F.E. session, while others attended multiple sessions. In general, the results were more favorable from those clients who had more than one L.I.F.E. session. The following are the results:

- The average response to the question "Your overall satisfaction with the L.I.F.E. session(s) you received" was **4.4** (out of 5).
- The average response to the question "How effective were the sessions in alleviating your primary complaint/issue?" was **4.0**.
- The average response to the question "How relaxed were you after the session(s)?" was **4.8**.
- The average response to the question "How transformative were these session(s)?" was **3.6**. Perhaps the clients didn't quite understand what "transformative" meant in this context.
- The average response to the question "Would you recommend L.I.F.E. biofeedback to a friend?" was **4.5**.

Below are some of the verbatims received:

"It was amazing to me that this system could reveal my problems, the ones I knew about and ones I didn't know about, but suspected."

"The system revealed a former life that was very relevant to an experience and dream I had when visiting a certain historical site two years ago."

"Several of my family members and I had several L.I.F.E. virtual sessions (as we live in Europe) and every time this system has proven to be accurate and effective. The system provided me with profound insights about my unconscious emotional problems, which caused dysfunctions and imbalances in my physical body. Some of these issues were related to events from past lives, while others were rooted in events from this life. I don't know if I would have been able to identify these emotional issues on my own, or how long it would have taken me, but the solutions, recommendations and energy balancing that the L.I.F.E. system provided were very effective and helped me a great deal. I was surprised that I could sense the energy in real time, even though the sessions were happening during the night and I was asleep at that time. The energy sent by L.I.F.E. was so powerful that I would wake up feeling engulfed in a very pleasant, beneficial energy, healing me on many levels. Out of all healing modalities I have tried so far, the L.I.F.E. system is the most effective, being able to diagnose, as well treat, many issues. Everybody in my family has greatly benefitted from these sessions."

"Overall it was enjoyable and very relaxing. I did not know what to expect. I think I would need more sessions to really evaluate if it has impact to my situation. On the other hand it may be working on things in the background and away from my awareness."

"Very effective for my menstrual pain - immediately felt better."

"My 14-year old dog had many health issues, mostly related to the heart and spleen, which caused him to be very lethargic and not able to walk or stand. The vet advised us to put him to sleep, given his age and his many health issues, including what the vet suspected as cancer, based on the results of a spleen tomography. However, we could not accept this outcome and asked Andrea for a L.I.F.E. session. The result was amazing! Our dear dog became his old self again, started to move, eat and go outdoors. It was obvious that his health had suddenly returned to him. At the next visit, the vet was very surprised of the tomography results: our dog's spleen was now almost normal in size and functioning well for his age. Same with his heart! It's been months now, but our dog is still in good health."

"This was just one session, but there was some impact, similar to the QXCI [another quantum biofeedback device]."

"After the L.I.F.E. treatment my condition improved, but not completely. Perhaps [my hearing impairment and dizziness]

was caused by a trauma, or an obstruction of a blood vessel in the right inner ear. At any rate, I feel that my recovery has been aided by the biofeedback sessions."

"The L.I.F.E. session was amazing. I am very sensitive to energy and I could sense how the system was scanning me and working on me, sending me energy, starting with the crown chakra and ending with the soles of my feet. I could sense different energy going to different parts of my body. At some point it felt like thousands of small needles working all over my body, and though intense, it was also very pleasant. I would repeat this wonderful L.I.F.E. session anytime and recommend it to others. After the session, I felt that all my chakras and meridians were balanced, and even now, though several months have passed since the session, I still feel very good."

"I think the sessions are amazing in that the electromagnetic field can be read and manipulated to create healing and balance. I believe the more consistent the sessions, the better the results. When I was going often, I felt better, had less pain. The environment is very comfortable and I have confidence in the therapist."

"I could clearly feel the energy/energetic transformation within my body as Andrea began using the various diagnostic panels for energy balancing/healing (a heightened awareness of the bigger earth school picture; a pronounced sense of calm & well being; dissipated anxiety and depression as a result of

the chronic stress that I am under due to my husband's cancer; reduction of fear and anger; relief from daily repetitive coughing episodes; a reduction of widespread inflammation throughout my physical body; the shedding of old behaviors; and a clearer picture/the ability to 'remember' the purpose for our time here by tuning into the collective consciousness). My session time flies by. I feel healthier, physically less clogged up, emotionally more balanced. I've also found the past life regressions that Andrea facilitated to be most helpful. Being regressed to a previous lifetime (that I would say seems to be the root cause of continued issues with my mother over the past several hundred years, as well as my subsequent molestation in my most recent past) has helped me to gain a more holistic understanding of my interaction with my family. Having this information has helped to encourage me to begin to work through the lessons that I've been struggling with in 'this time,' so as to change the past and present outcome(s), by energetically re-scripting them, thereby affording me the ability to heal in all dimensions. The L.I.F.E. system's ability to pinpoint 'life event' issues (without assistance from the subject) was also remarkable. Its diagnostic capability to pinpoint, by the subject's age and surrounding event/s, energetic issues being stored in the body from that 'trauma' shows us that there are many forms of muscle memory. This roadmap has helped me to remember the event(s) that I had otherwise forgotten and needed to clear/balance. I am a 61 year old female and the identified issues were from when I was 8 and 34 years old."

Conclusions

After working with the L.I.F.E. system for two years now, I strongly believe that it's very effective in identifying stress factors and relieving stress -- physical, emotional, mental and spiritual. The system is often accurate in identifying a client's most pressing issues and the majority of clients have reported feeling very relaxed and refreshed after a session. Some clients have insightful recollections of traumatic events in their life, and the sessions allow them to process these and heal. Many clients feel the beneficial energies sent by the system, in the form of tingles, vibrations, or temperature changes. Each biofeedback session is unique, because the client's body guides the session according to its own wisdom. Many clients observe improvements to their condition after 2-3 sessions, though some see drastic results right away. I can't explain why some clients see immediate benefits, while others don't, but it may be related to their desire to heal. Some people might say they want to heal, but unconsciously they don't, as they reap emotional benefits from being sick (e.g., getting more attention, love, etc.).

I counsel my clients to lead a healthy lifestyle, exercise regularly, eat a healthy diet and strive to keep balance between body, mind and spirit, as Edgar Cayce advised. Healing involves shifting *mental and emotional* patterns, and the L.I.F.E. system enables that beautifully. Cayce also believed that circulation, assimilation, relaxation, and elimination are the keys to healing, wellness, and longevity, and again the L.I.F.E. system can help balance these four items. I strongly encourage my clients to take personal responsibility for their healing and wellbeing. Cayce compares illness with a musical instrument that's out of tune (Reading 317-7). When our vibrations are adjusted/balanced properly, we experience healing.

There are many opportunities for further research with the L.I.F.E. system, ideally if conducted by licensed doctors, dentists and psychologists. Some potential research ideas would be to determine the efficacy of the L.I.F.E. system on clients suffering from migraines, allergies, depression, anxiety, Lyme disease, AIDS and cancer. Perhaps the Rife community may also be interested in researching the L.I.F.E. system, as it includes many "Rife-like" frequencies. I personally would like to explore more the **Timed/Specific Panel**, where I could enter specific Rife frequencies from the Rife Handbook (Sylver, 2011, ch. 5).

I have come to think of the L.I.F.E. system as a "consciousness device," involving the consciousness of the practitioner and the client, engaged in the sacred dance of healing. With the help of the L.I.F.E. system, clients can expand their consciousness, deepen their awareness and transform spiritually. There are some wonderfully uplifting frequencies for Ascendance, Astral Projection, Clairvoyance, ESP Stimulation, Meditation Stimulation, Mystical Stimulation, Past Life Regression, Shaman State, Transcendence, and Unity with All. From my experience, when these frequencies are applied regularly, they accelerate a client's spiritual evolution. This strikes to the core of my mission in this lifetime, which is to accelerate the evolution of consciousness.

I am honored to be one of the few L.I.F.E. System practitioners in the United States and I'm looking forward to helping many clients achieve the highest levels of wellbeing.

References

Amoroso, J. (2012). *Awakening past lives. A step-by-step guide to self-explorations*. Virginia Beach, VA: 4th Dimension Press.

Baud, W., & Anderson, R. (1998). *Transpersonal research methods for the social sciences.* Thousand Oaks, CA: SAGE Publications, Inc.

Biofeedback. (2014). In *College for international holistic studies online*. Retrieved from http://www.naturalmedicinecollege.ca/diploma-programs/biofeedback-therapist/

Biofeedback Federation of Europe. (2014). In *Clinical protocols online.* Retrieved from http://bfe.org/new/news/protocols

Bradden, G. (2007). *The divine matrix. Bridging time, space, miracles and belief.* Carlsbad, CA: Hay House, Inc.

Cayce, E. (1971). *Edgar Cayce readings*. Virginia Beach: Edgar Cayce Foundation.

Chopra, D. (1989). *Quantum healing. Exploring the frontiers of mind/body medicine.* New York, NY: Bantam Books.

Cook, M. (2004). *The 4-week ultimate body detox plan*. Hoboken, NJ: John Wiley & Sons, Inc.

Hemi-Sync. (2014). In *The Monroe Institute online*. Retrieved from http://www.monroeinstitute.org/resources/hemi-sync

Henderson, L. (2009). *The history and guidelines of biofeedback.* Milton, Ontario: The College of International Holistic Studies.

Henderson, L. (2010). *Biofeedback level one manual.* Milton, Ontario: The College of International Holistic Studies.

L.I.F.E. Biofeedback System. (2013). In *L.I.F.E. System online.* Retrieved from http://www.lifesysteminternational.com/

Lynes, B. (2009). *Rife's world of electromedicine: The story, the corruption and the promise.* South Lake Tahoe, CA: BioMed Publishing Group.

National Center for Complementary and Alternative Medicine (NCCAM). (2014). In *Biofeedback search results online.* Retrieved from http://nccam.nih.gov

Rife, R. (2007). In *Research papers online.* Retrieved from http://www.rife.org/otherresearch.html

Sylver, N. (2011). *The Rife handbook of frequency therapy and holistic health.* South Lake Tahoe, CA: BioMed Publishing Group.

World Health Organization. (2010). In *Biofeedback search results online.* Retrieved from http://www.who.int/en/

Appendix A

L.I.F.E. System Technical Information (from the L.I.F.E. website)

The measurement made by the L.I.F.E. System is based upon the relationship between "action & reaction" by applying a challenge to the patient ("action") and measuring the reaction of the human body as it answers the challenge ("reaction").

The basic principle of the mode of action of the L.I.F.E. System device is the following: the L.I.F.E. System device sends a square wave signal with amplitude of 5 Volt, and a duty cycle of 50% to the harness. The frequency to be applied, for determination of our test, is about 47.3 kHz. The measurement current through the body is limited to a maximum of 10mA, but usually no more than 5mA or less.

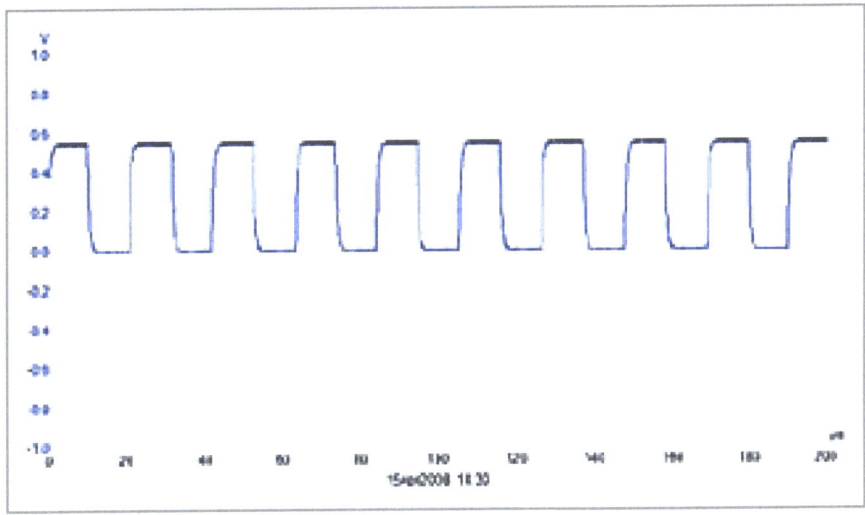

Figure 1: *Square wave signal with no harness in contact with the human body.*

When the harness is in contact with the human body, a significant change (deformation) of the signal can be detected. Figure 2 shows the respective signals (but on a different time scale to underline the changes).

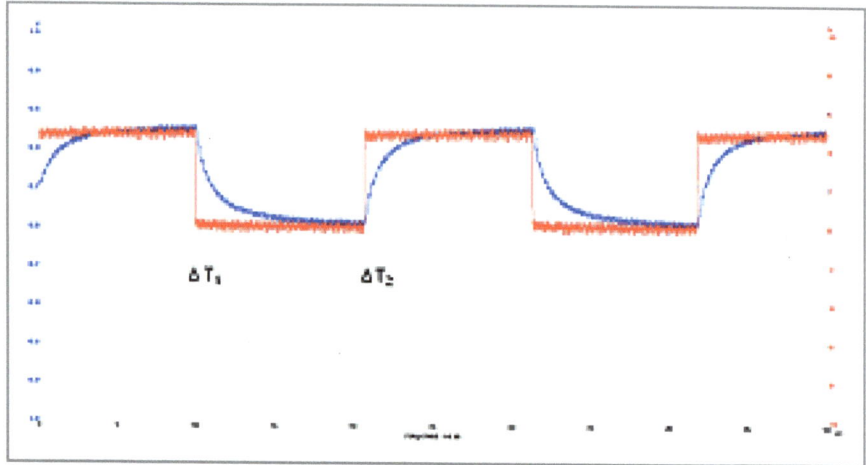

Figure 2: *Superimposition of the signal without harness being applied to the human body (red signal) and with electrodes being applied to the human body (blue signal).*

As can be seen from the superimposition of the signals, there is a significant difference in the shapes of the signals. The detection of the signal is realized by the L.I.F.E. System device in a binary way – the part of the signal being placed in the upper half of the square wave signal is detected, the lower part of the square wave signal is ignored. Therefore, the different shapes of the signals (electrodes applied to a patient and no electrodes applied to the patient) result in time differences $\Delta T1$ and $\Delta T2$ before half of the amplitude is passed. These time differences resulting from the

48

different shapes of the signals are detected by the L.I.F.E. System device.

When applying the same methodology to a patient suffering from a particular imbalance, again a signal will be detected. But as the situation in the body of the patient is different due to the imbalance, the shape of the signal to be detected is different, and it can be seen that this signal is less steep in the case of imbalance. This difference in signal shapes results in other time differences Δt1 and Δt2, which are characteristic for a particular imbalance.

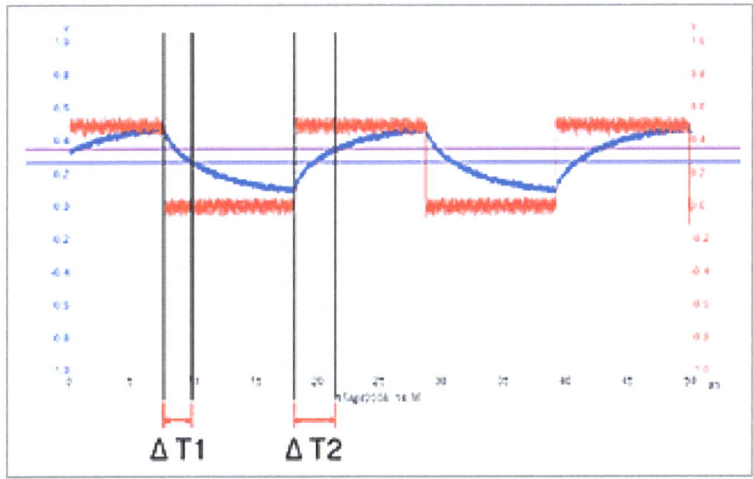

Figure 3: Superimposing the signal obtained from a patient suffering from a particular imbalance (blue signal) and the signal obtained when harness is not applied to the human body (red signal).

However, it must be pointed out that the results obtained by the L.I.F.E. System device can only give hints to physical states in which the presence of a particular imbalance is likely. The final diagnosis must be confirmed by other methodologies such as X-ray or MRI in any case.

The basic principle of the L.I.F.E. System device is to measure these time differences of the respective signals and to achieve a statistical evaluation based on a mathematical algorithm. The results obtained are compared with data which are archived in a data base.

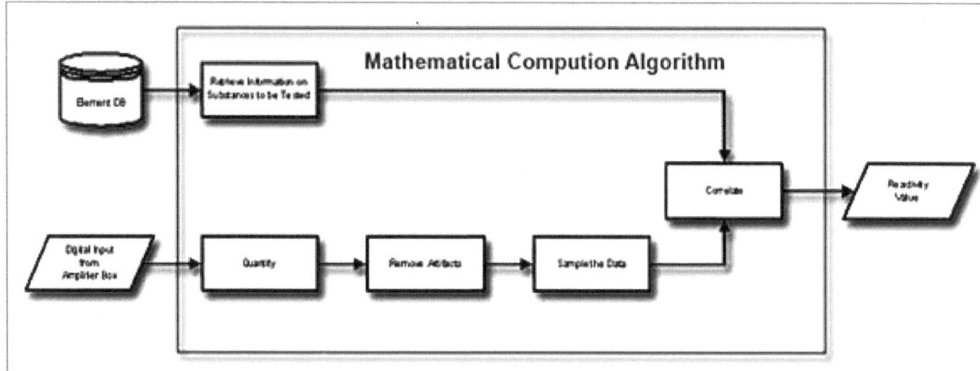

Figure 4: *Basic work flow for the evaluation of data obtained.*

The mathematical calculation algorithm takes input information on the one hand, which is stored in the Element database, and on the other hand the digitized measurement data, belonging to the element. After quantifying the values, artifacts (like disturbances caused by EMC, movements, etc.) are removed. The cleaned data is sampled and after that, the correlation is calculated, leading to the desired reactivity value, providing the results of reactivity testing, relative to the given element.

It can be claimed that when the situation inside the human body is disturbed due to a particular imbalance, the physical situation will become different. Any abnormal condition can be considered as a kind of imbalance. As a consequence, the shape of the signal that is detected will differ from the one measured in a non-conditional situation. The differences can be measured easily by detecting the time difference, as described above, and those time differences are characteristic for the respective situations. Evidence that they can be measured and detected was given by the outcome of the clinical investigation, which was undertaken in 2006.

Appendix B

Biofeedback Research

According to the National Center for Complementary and Alternative Medicine (NCCAM), the Biofeedback Federation of Europe (BFE) and the World Health Organization (WHO), there is ample research to prove that biofeedback is effective in treating fibromyalgia, headaches, stress, rheumatoid arthritis, chronic pain, diabetes, cancer and smoking addiction. On their website, BFE lists several clinical studies developed by major contributors in the field of biofeedback and physical therapy. These studies show that the use of electromyography (a form of biofeedback) is an effective tool for physiotherapy. Studies listed include Patellofemoral Pain Syndrome, Unstable Shoulder, Post-operative Knee, Urinary and Fecal Incontinence, Phantom Limb Pain, Chronic Tension Headache, Repetitive Strain Injury, among others.

The Royal Rife website lists several research papers describing the efficacy of the Rife frequencies on various diseases, including cancer. There is also a long list of lab reports from the Rife Research Laboratory, describing the experiments of applying various Rife frequencies on carcinoma, diphtheria, typhoid fever, tuberculosis, etc. Several related patents are also listed on this website.

According to the L.I.F.E. website, "literature in peer reviewed journals describing the mode of action and effectiveness" of quantum biofeedback was not available prior to the development of the L.I.F.E. System. Consequently, a "clinical investigation giving evidence to the effectiveness was undertaken in 2006. The complete documentation and the results have been submitted to and approved for European Class 2-A Certification. Rigorous testing, double-blind studies and subsequent approval by TUV Germany guarantee quality and efficacy."

Appendix C -- L.I.F.E. System Screen Prints

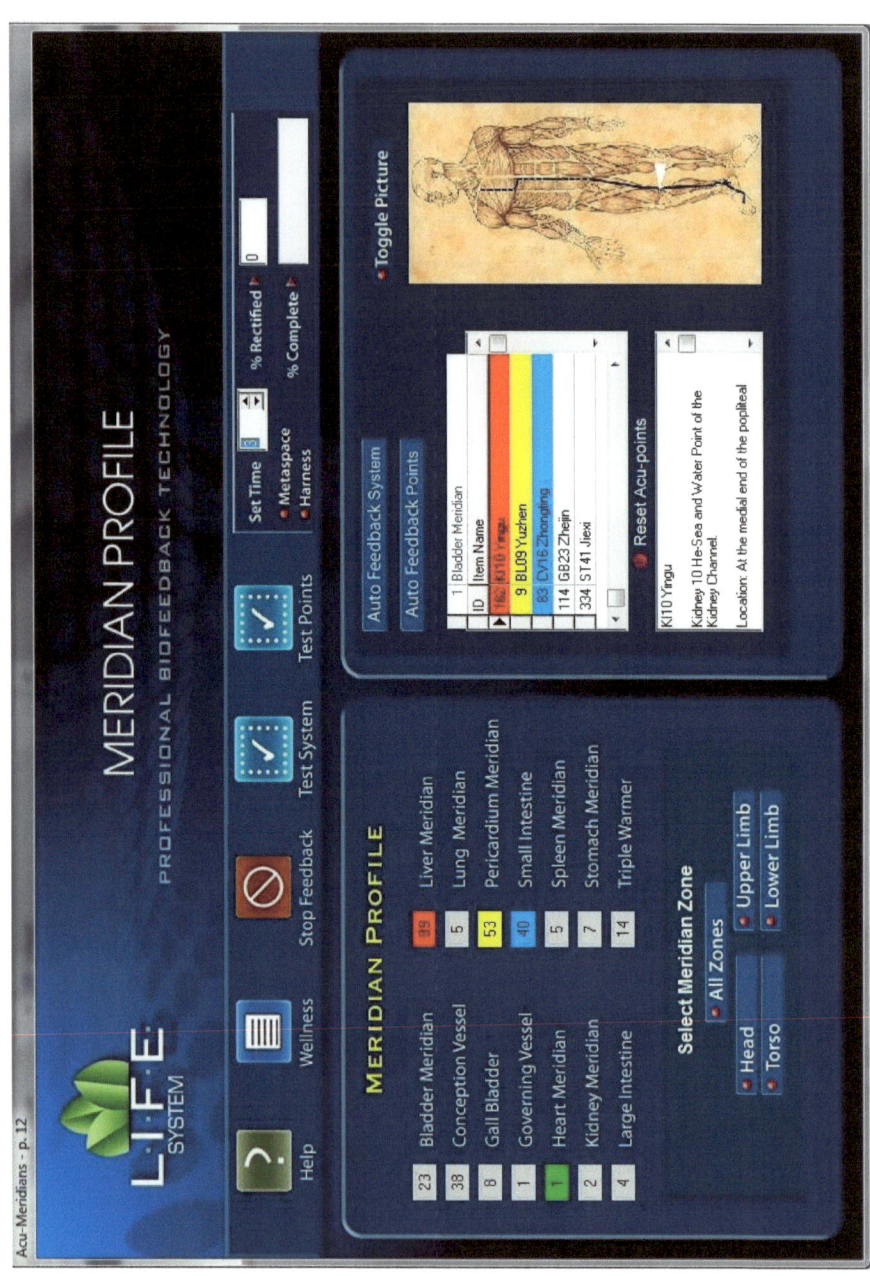

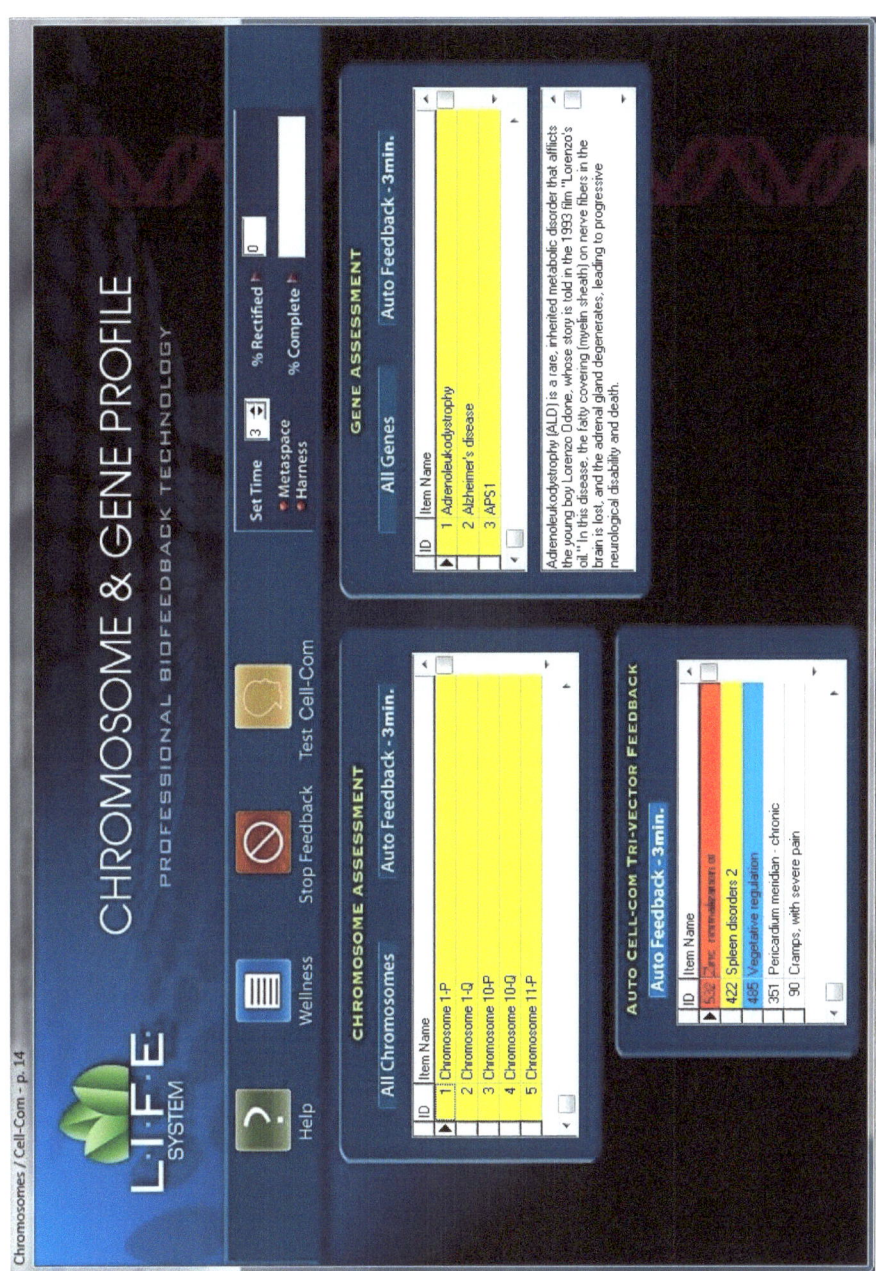

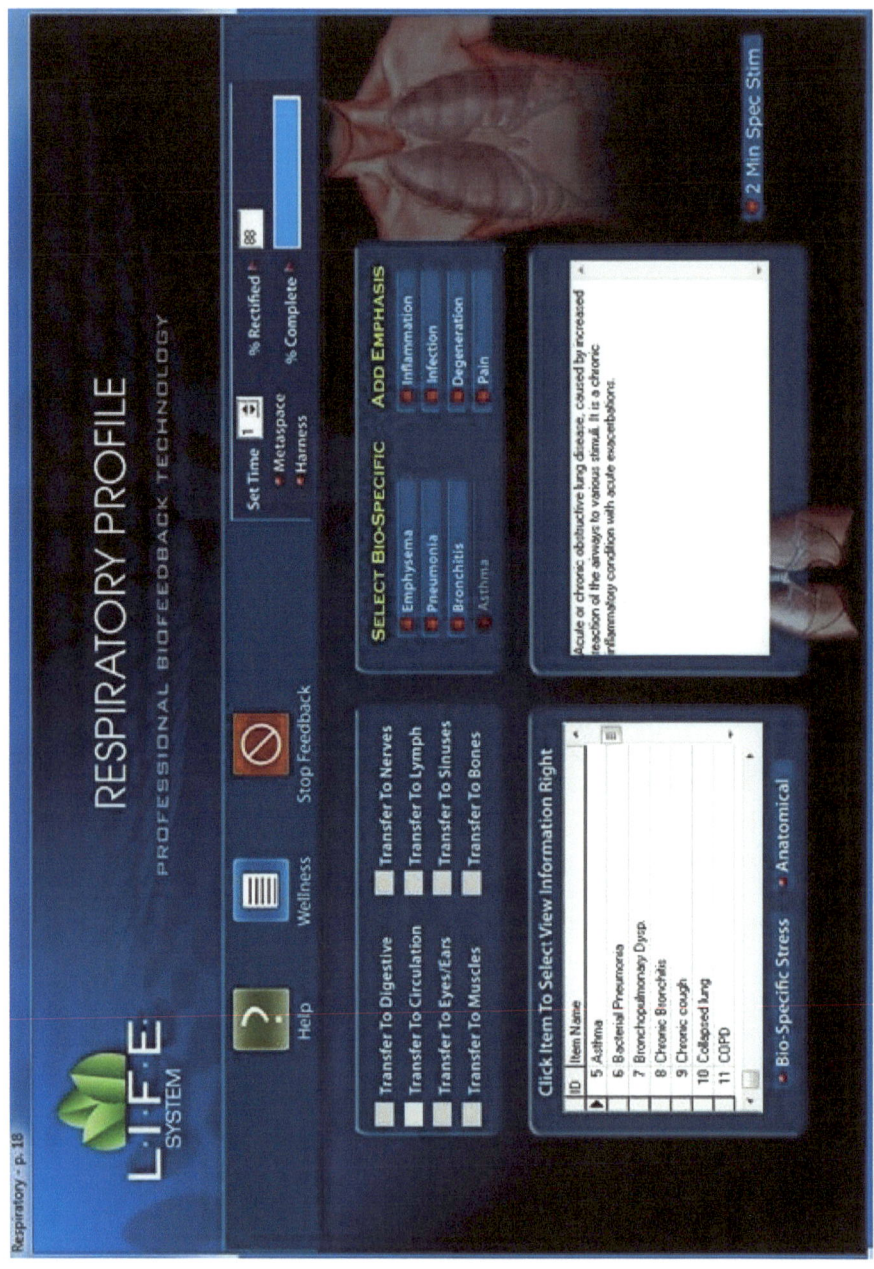

Respiratory - p. 18

RESPIRATORY PROFILE
PROFESSIONAL BIOFEEDBACK TECHNOLOGY

L·I·F·E SYSTEM

Help   Wellness   Stop Feedback

Transfer To Digestive   Transfer To Nerves
Transfer To Circulation   Transfer To Lymph
Transfer To Eyes/Ears   Transfer To Sinuses
Transfer To Muscles   Transfer To Bones

Set Time 1
• Metaspace   % Rectified
• Harness   % Complete   88

SELECT BIO-SPECIFIC   **ADD EMPHASIS**
• Emphysema   • Inflammation
• Pneumonia   • Infection
• Bronchitis   • Degeneration
• Asthma   • Pain

Acute or chronic obstructive lung disease, caused by increased reaction of the airways to various stimuli. It is a chronic inflammatory condition with acute exacerbations.

Click Item To Select View Information Right

ID	Item Name
5	Asthma
6	Bacterial Pneumonia
7	Bronchopulmonary Dysp.
8	Chronic Bronchitis
9	Chronic cough
10	Collapsed lung
11	COPD

• Bio-Specific Stress   • Anatomical

• 2 Min Spec Stim

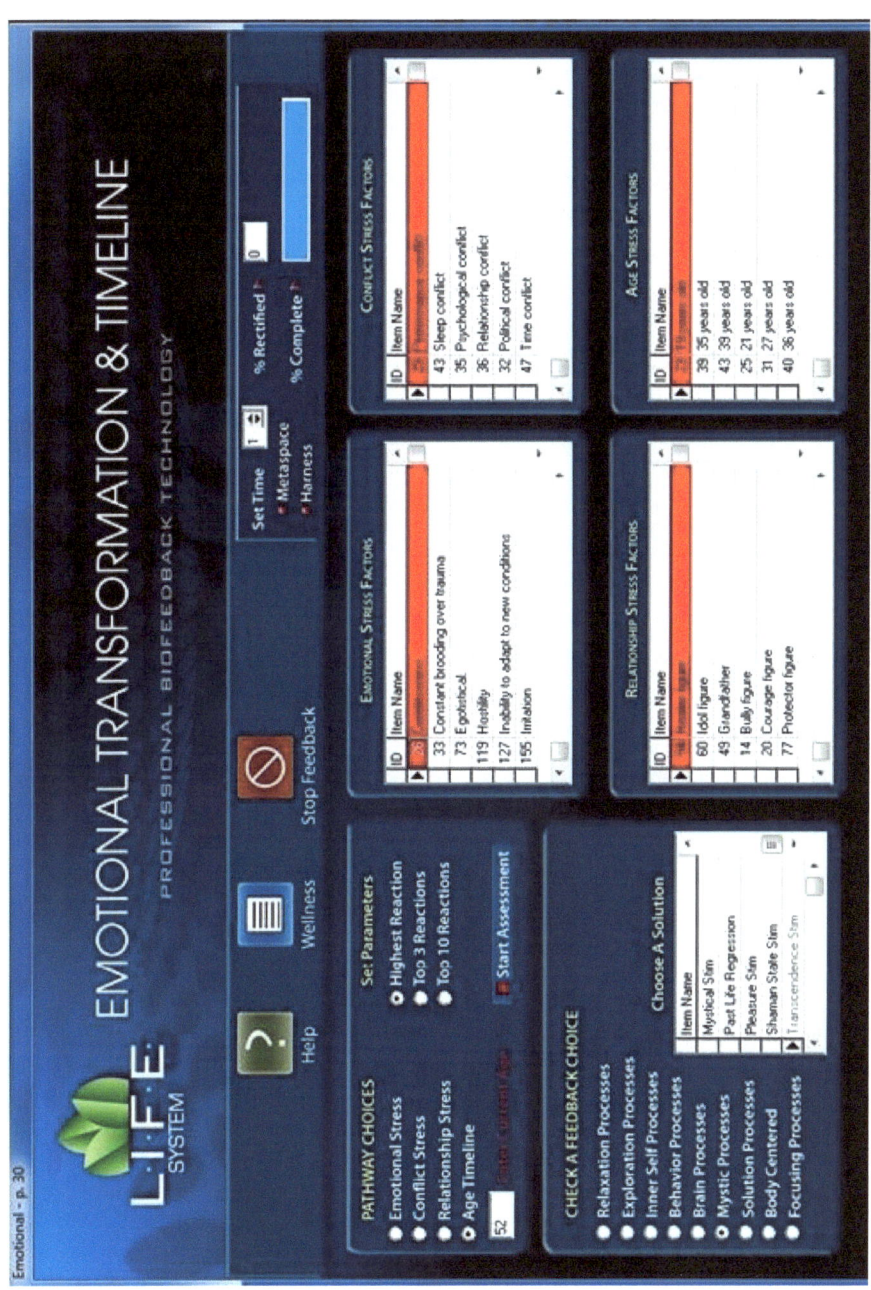

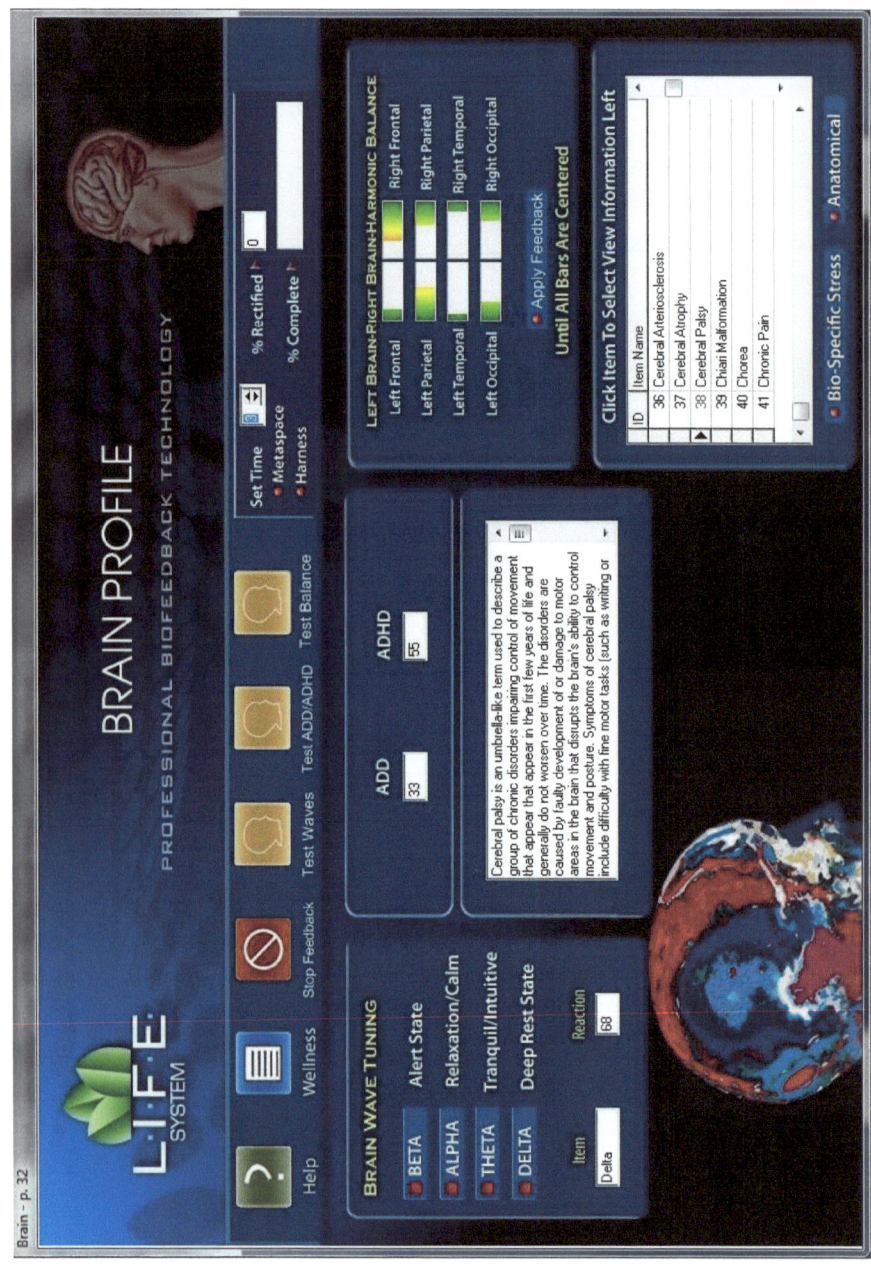

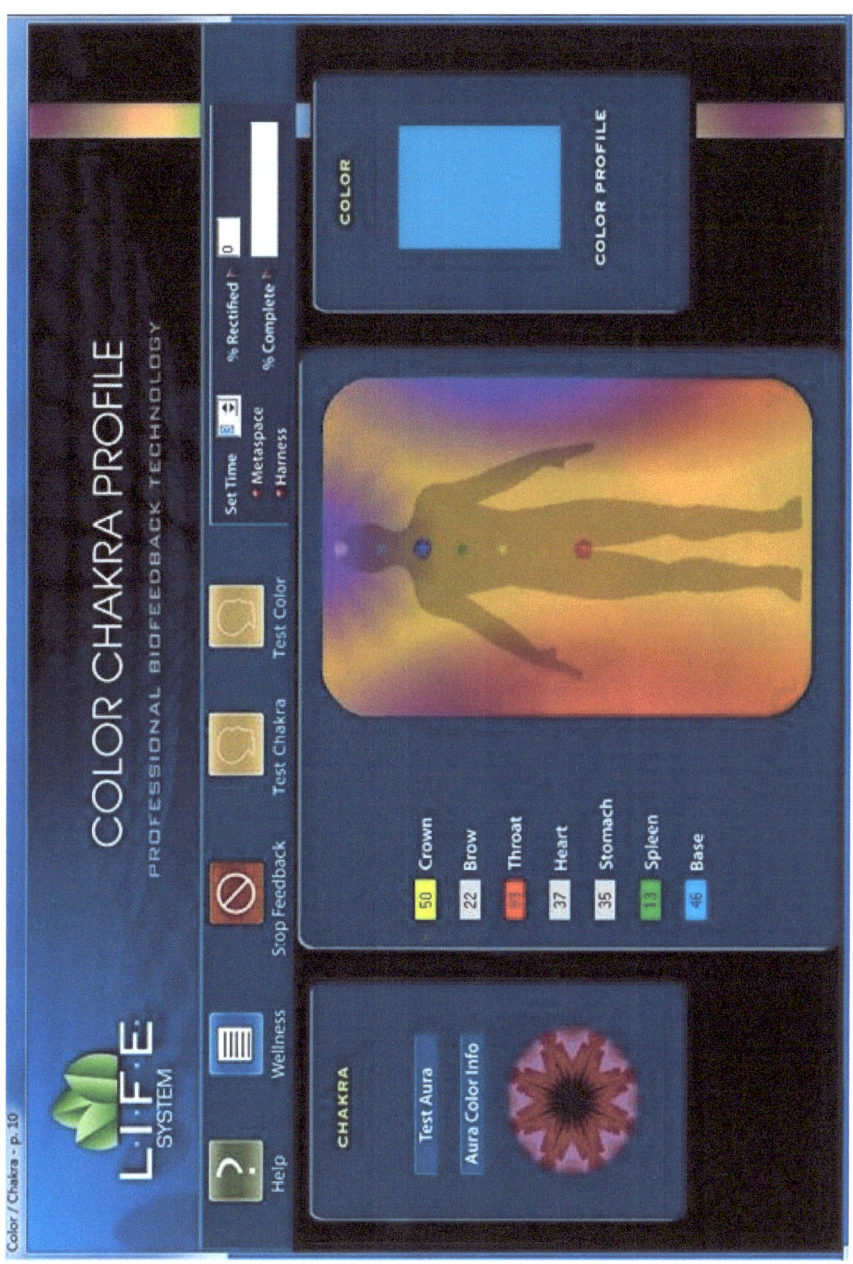

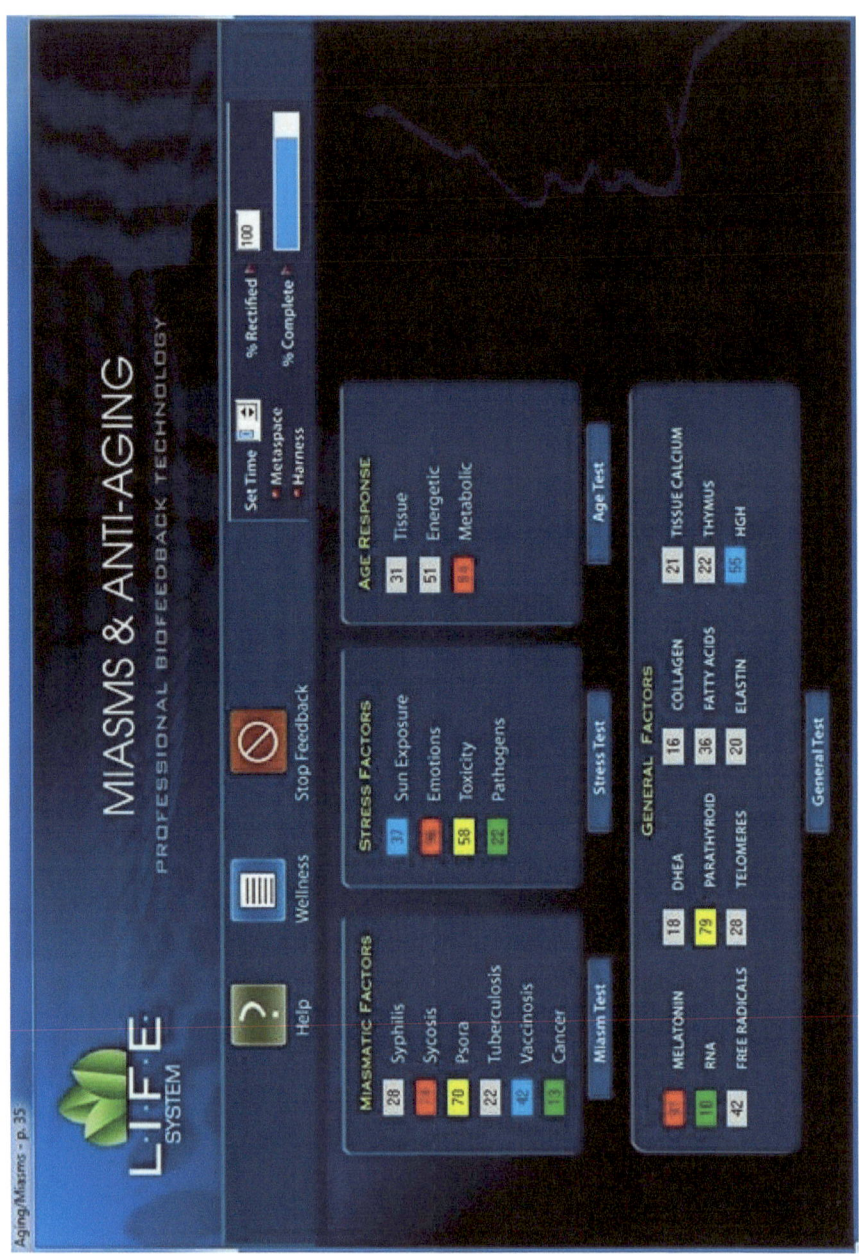

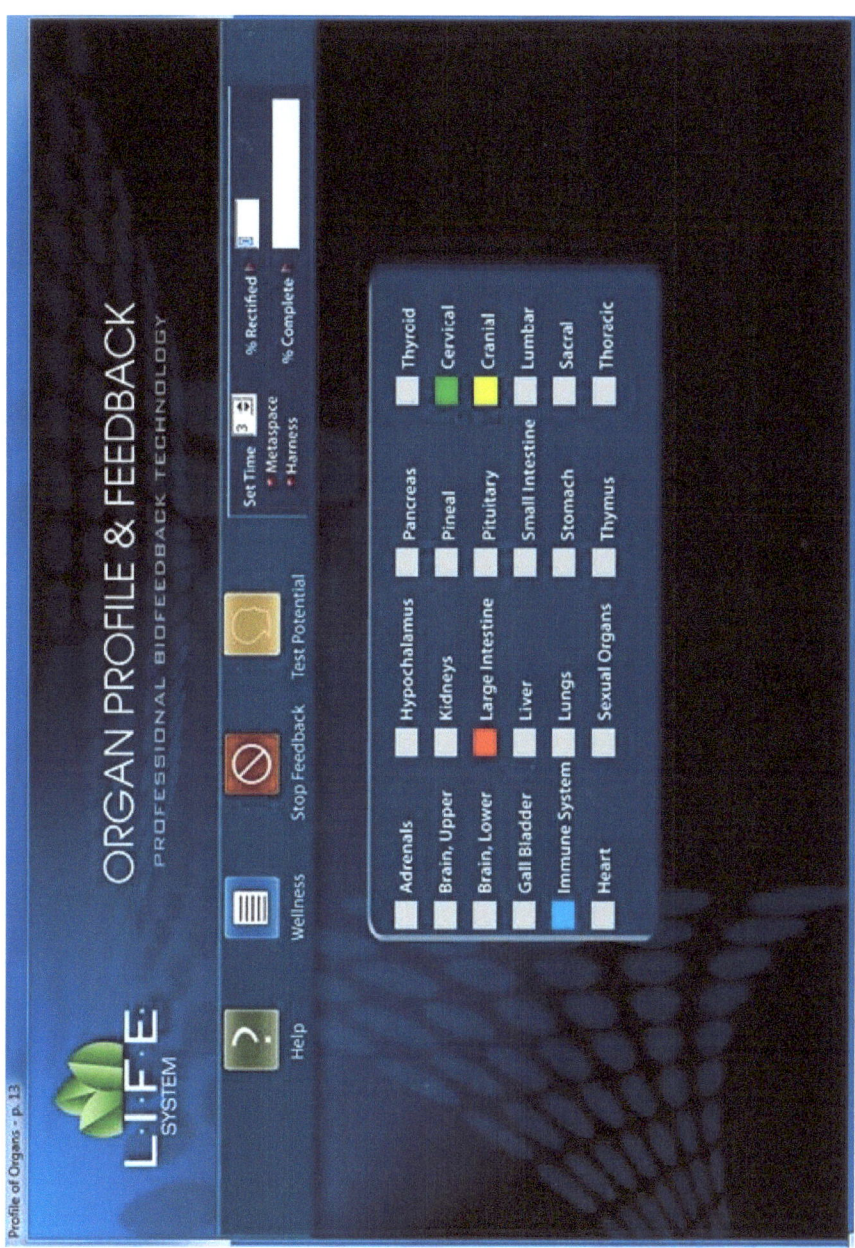

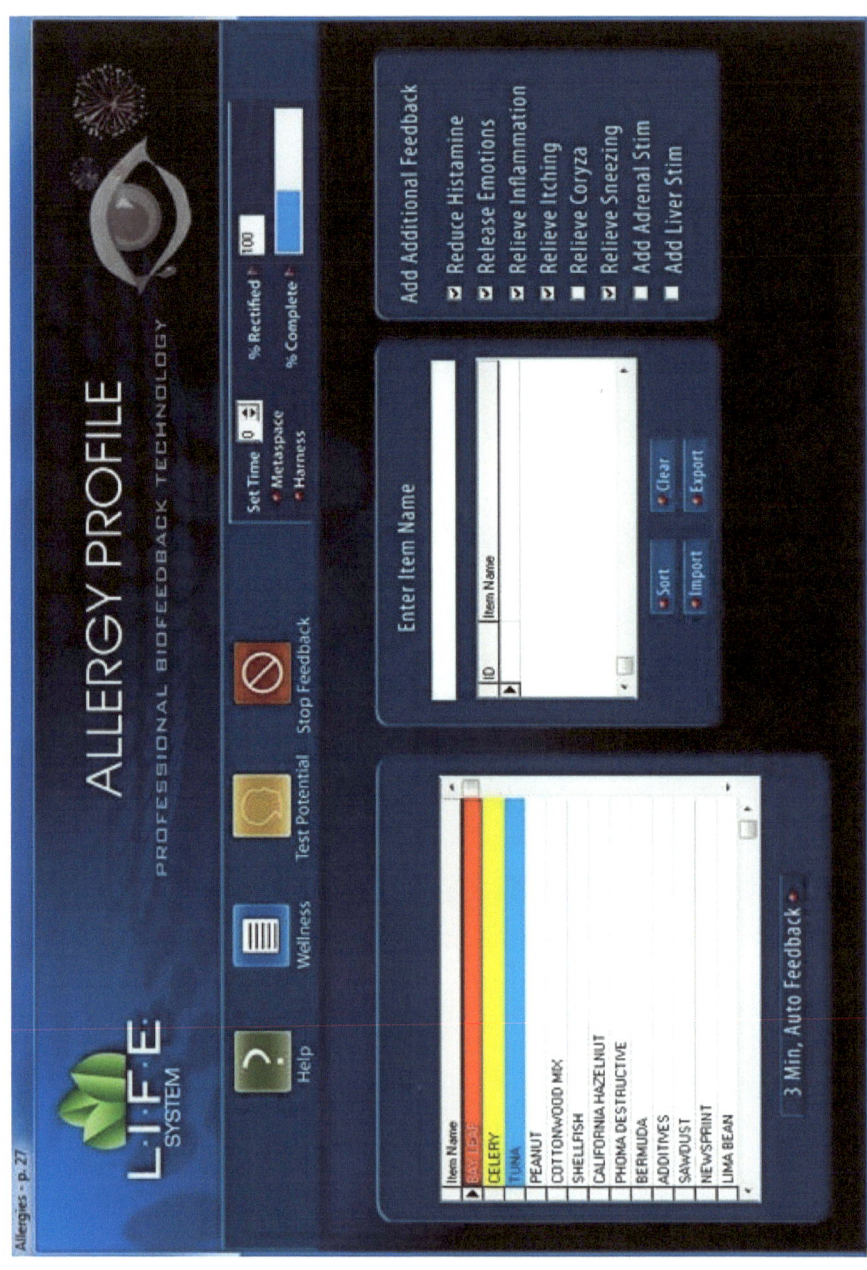

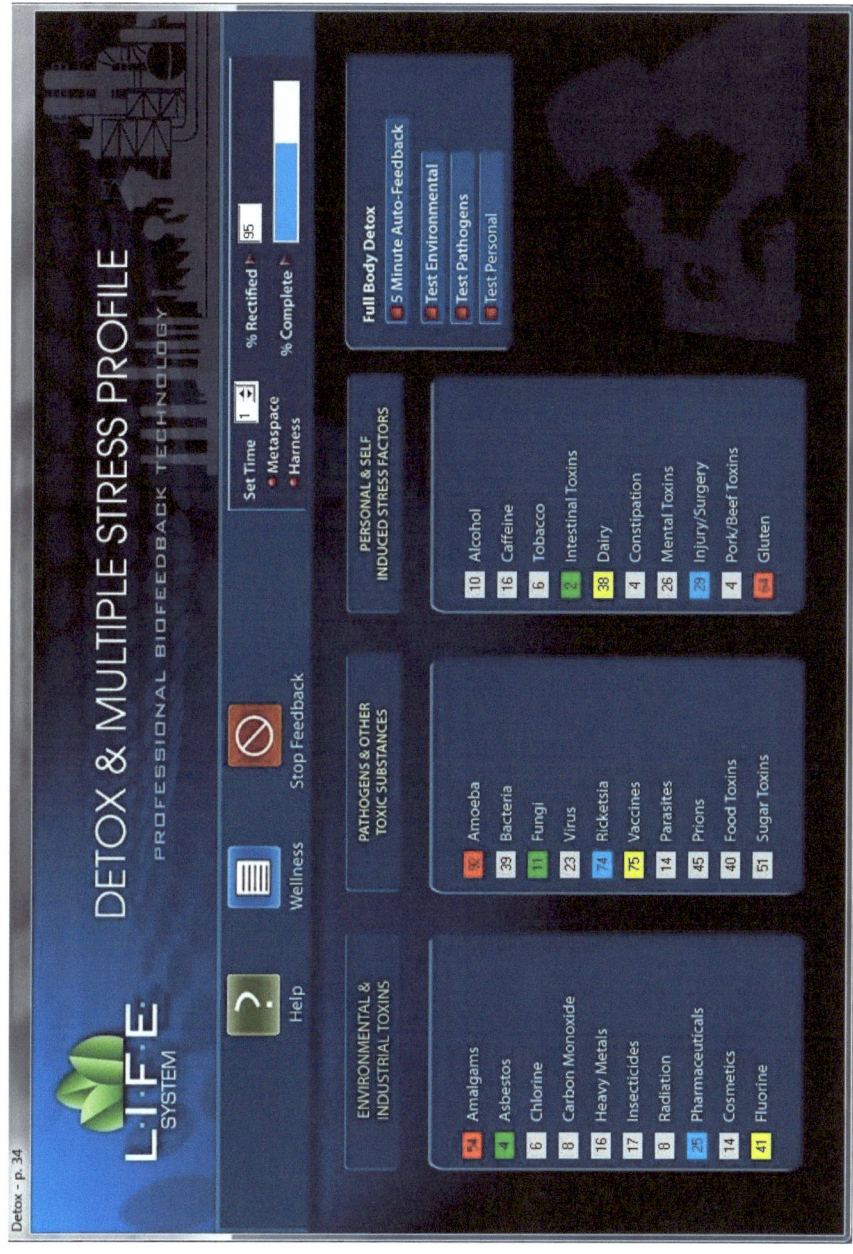

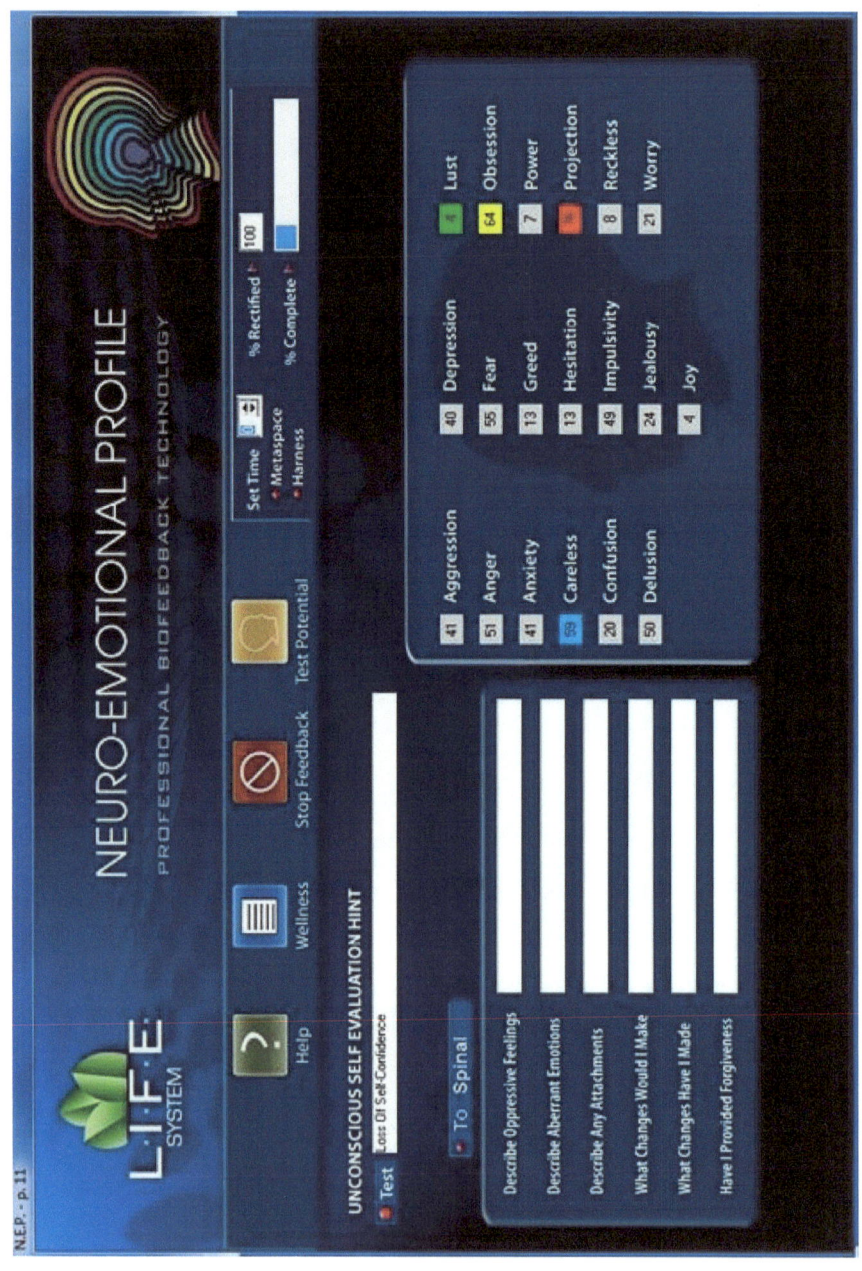

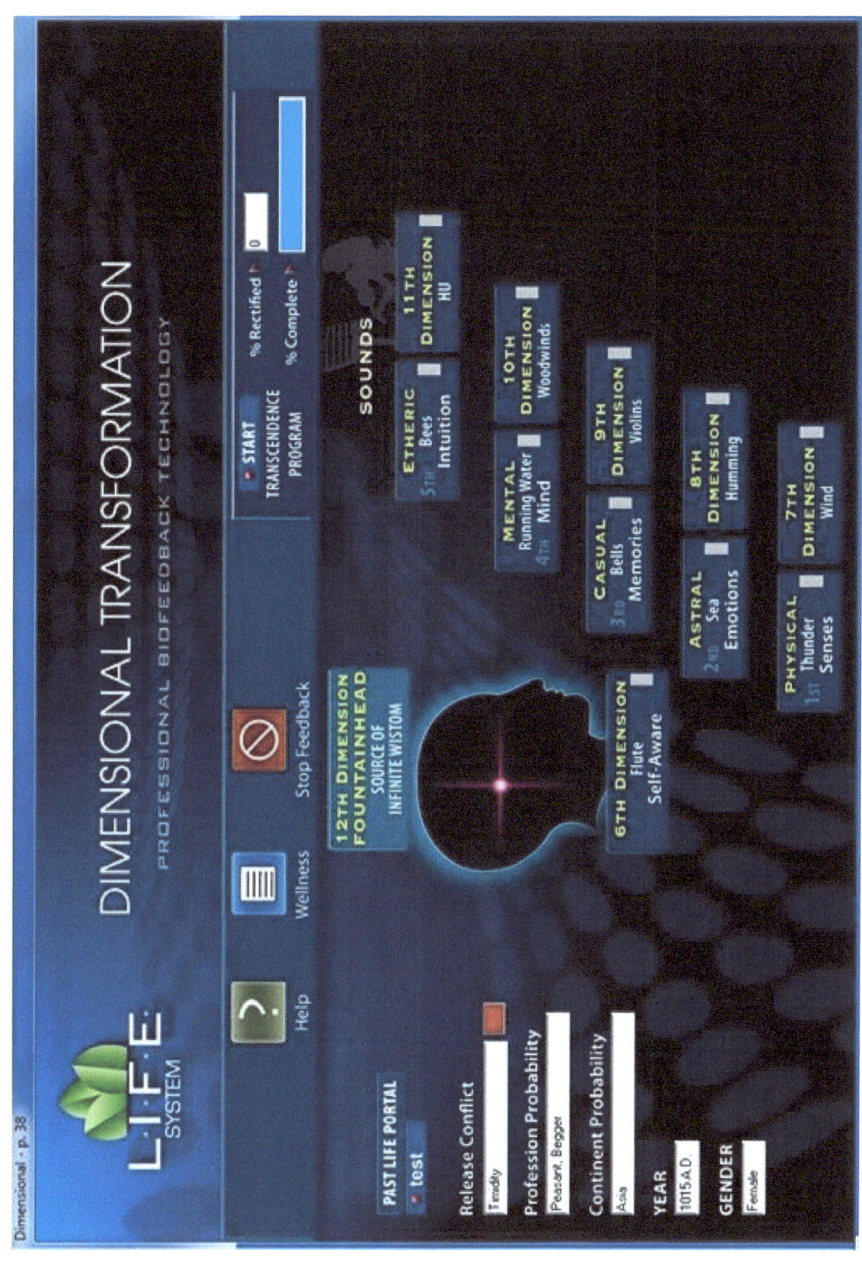

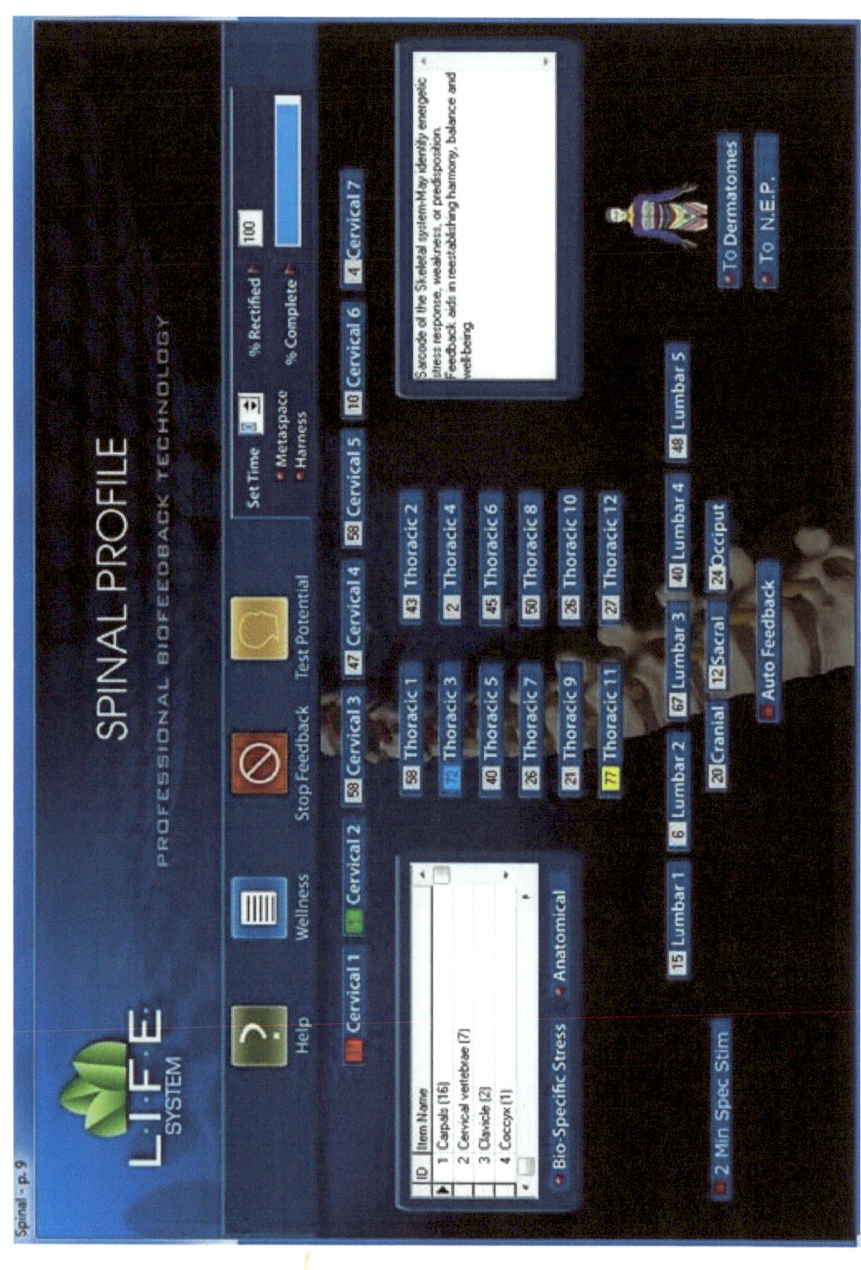

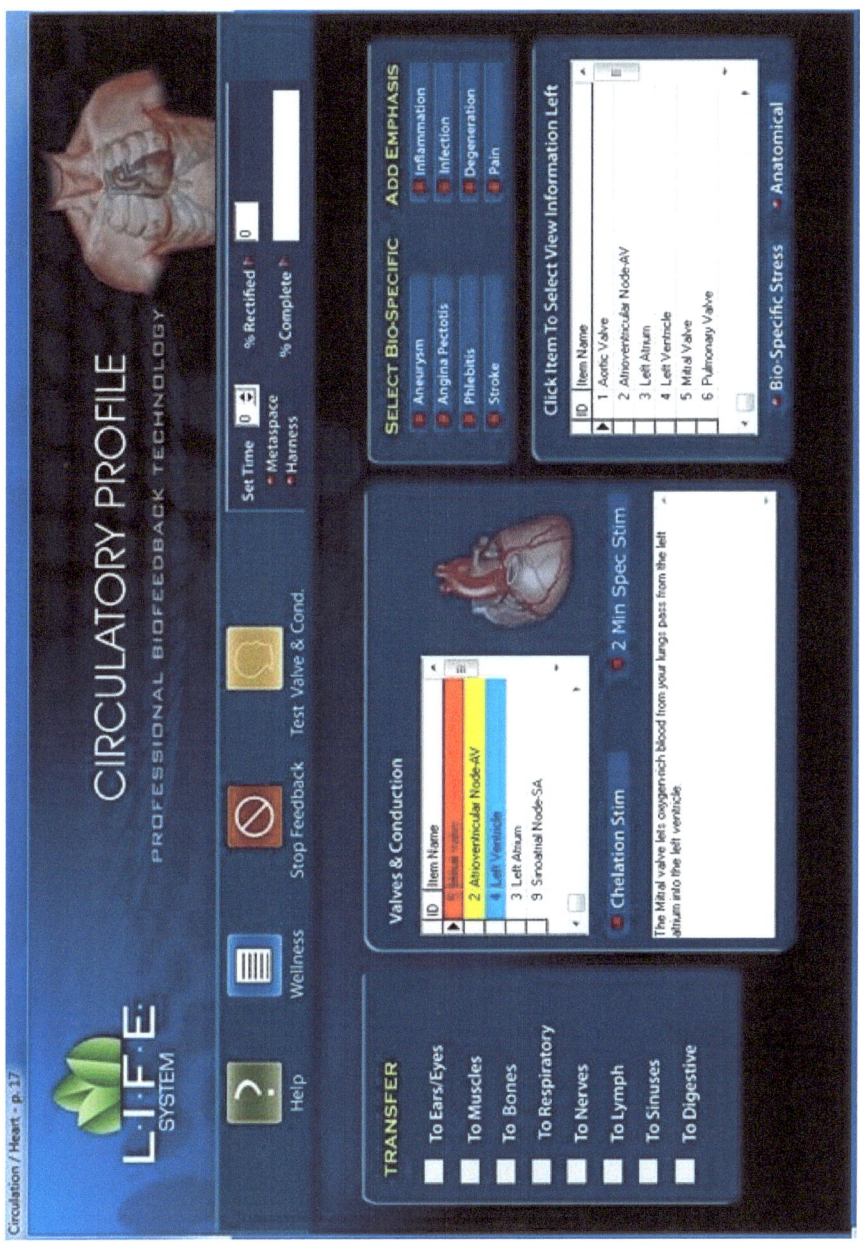

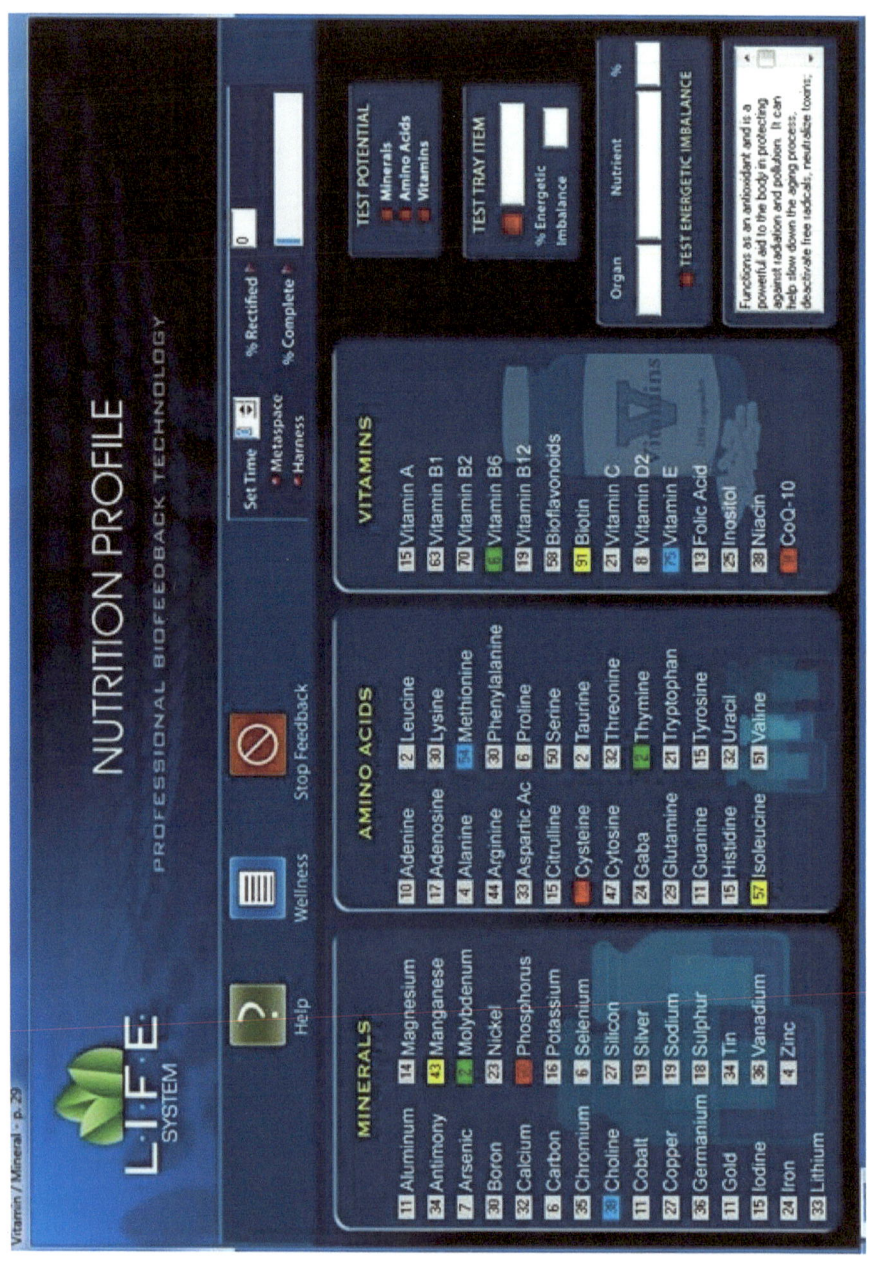

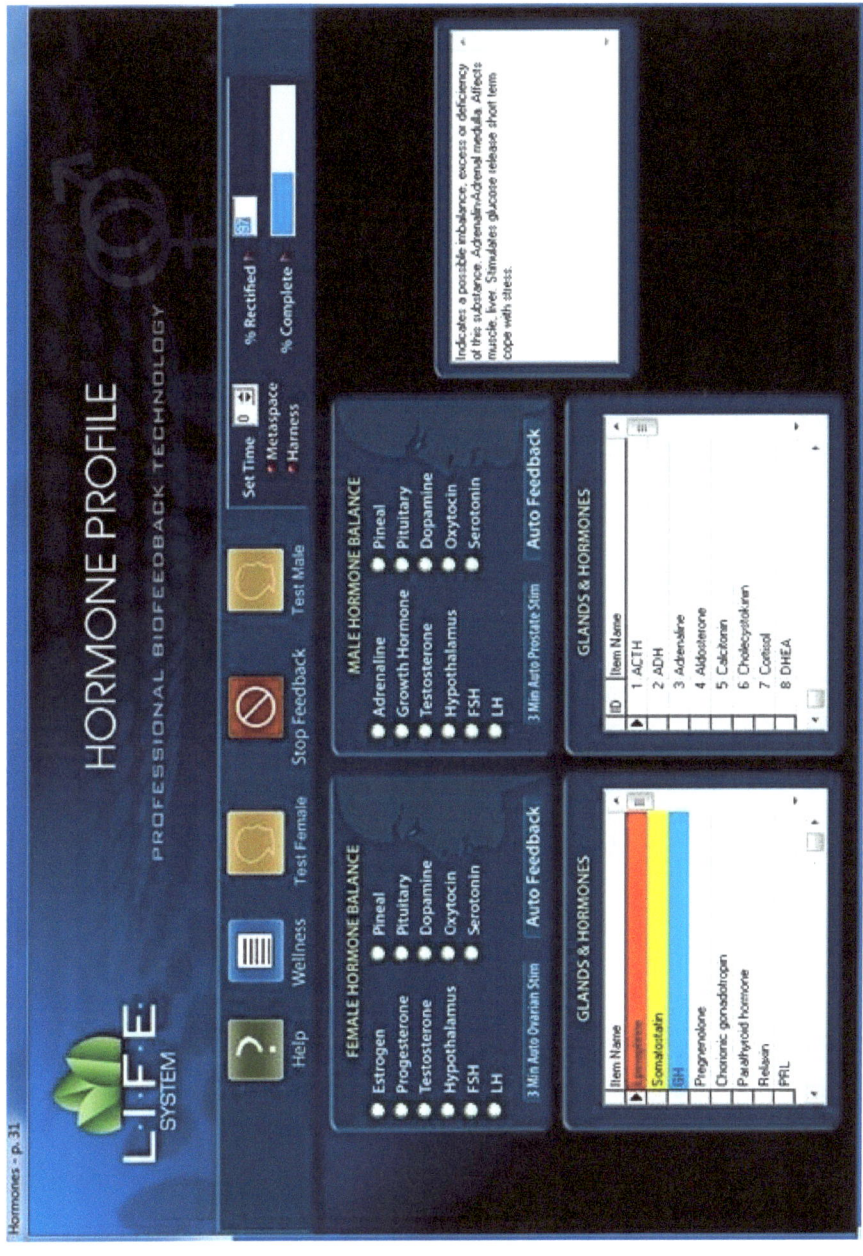

HORMONE PROFILE

PROFESSIONAL BIOFEEDBACK TECHNOLOGY

L·I·F·E·
SYSTEM

Help   Wellness   Test Female   Stop Feedback   Test Male

Set Time   0

• Metaspace
• Harness

% Rectified
% Complete

FEMALE HORMONE BALANCE

Estrogen   Pineal
Progesterone   Pituitary
Testosterone   Dopamine
Hypothalamus   Oxytocin
FSH   Serotonin
LH

3 Min Auto Ovarian Stim   Auto Feedback

MALE HORMONE BALANCE

Adrenaline   Pineal
Growth Hormone   Pituitary
Testosterone   Dopamine
Hypothalamus   Oxytocin
FSH   Serotonin
LH

3 Min Auto Prostate Stim   Auto Feedback

GLANDS & HORMONES

Item Name
Somatostatin
Somatostatin
GH
Pregnenolone
Chorionic gonadotropin
Parathyroid hormone
Relaxin
PRL

GLANDS & HORMONES

ID	Item Name
1	ACTH
2	ADH
3	Adrenaline
4	Aldosterone
5	Calcitonin
6	Cholecystokinin
7	Cortisol
8	DHEA

Indicates a possible imbalance, excess or deficiency of this substance. Adrenalin-Adrenal medulla. Affects muscle, liver. Stimulates glucose release short term cope with stress.

69

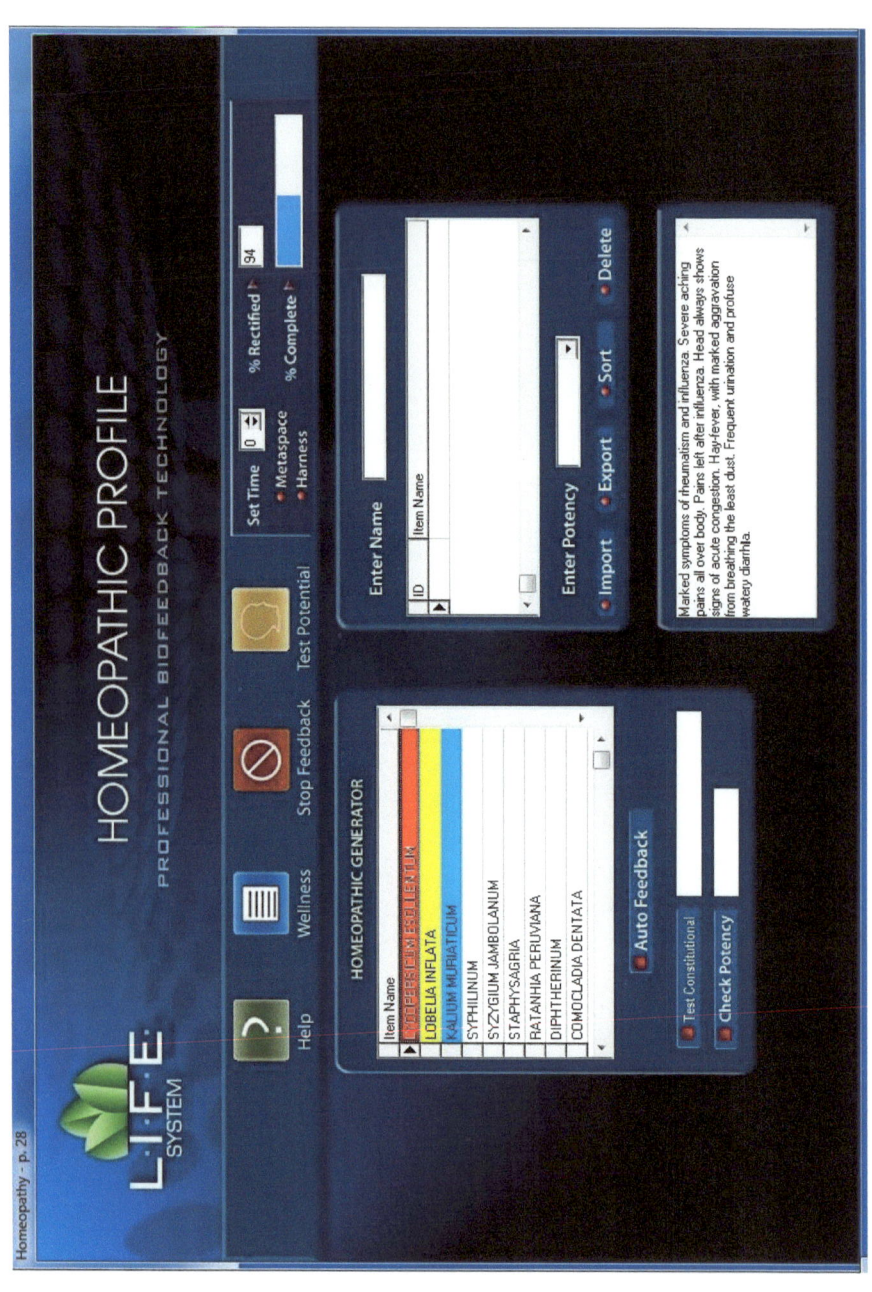

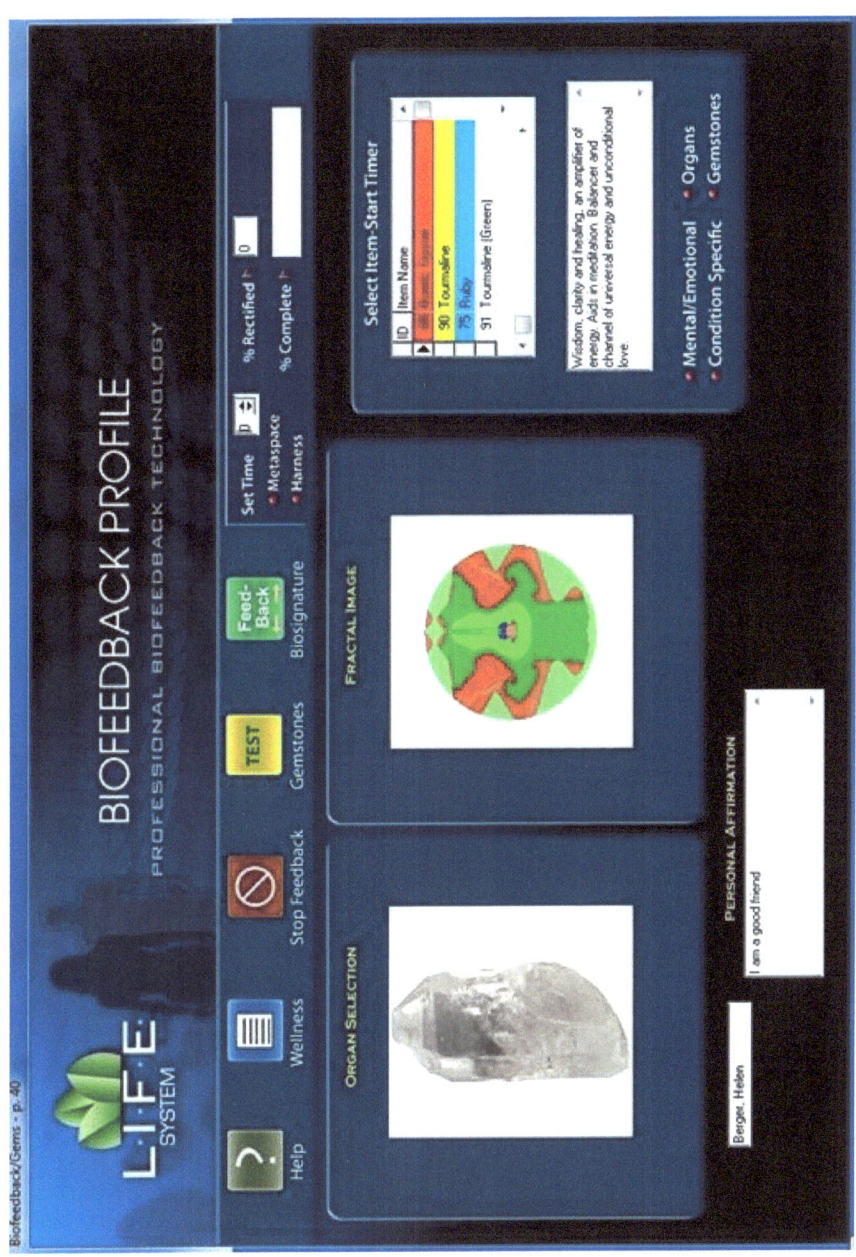

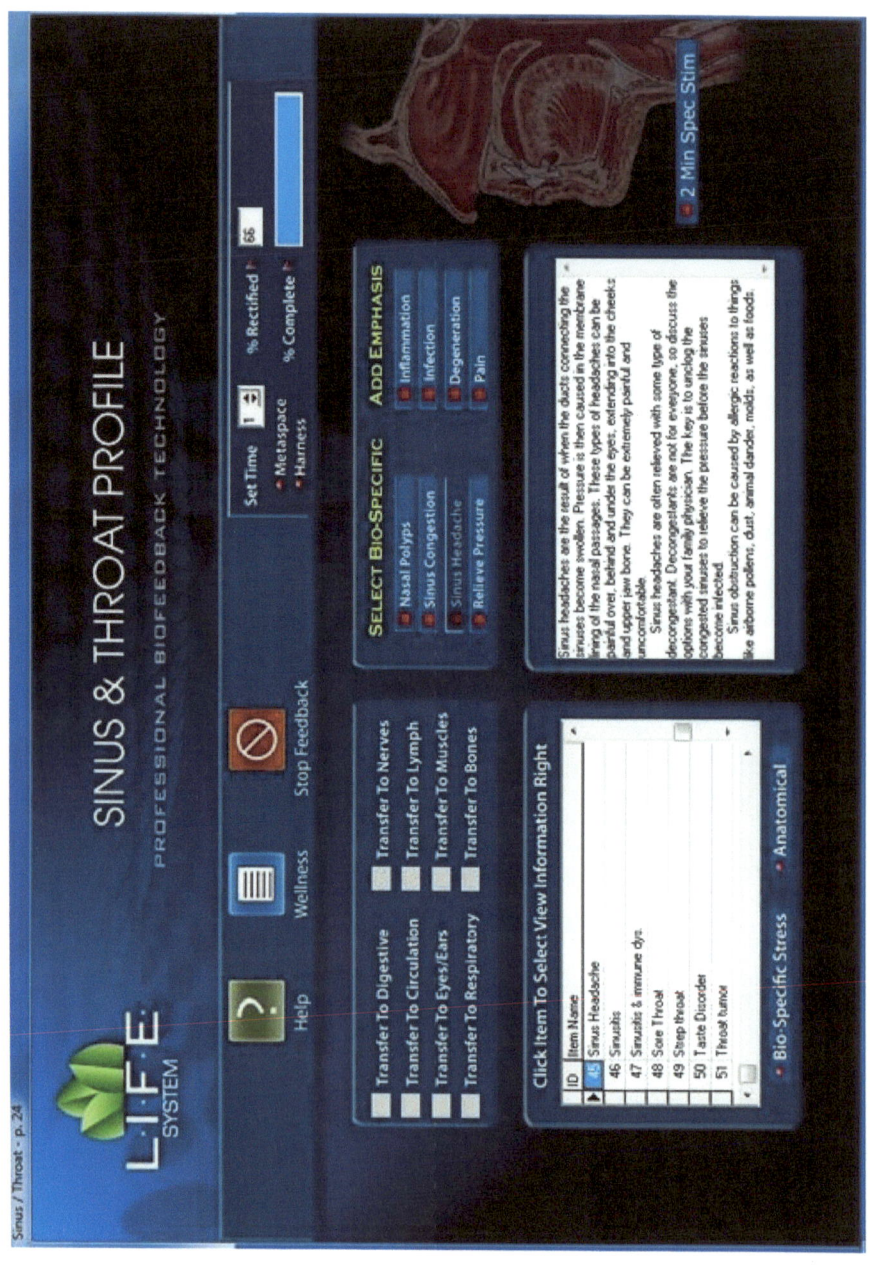

SINUS & THROAT PROFILE

PROFESSIONAL BIOFEEDBACK TECHNOLOGY

Help   Wellness   Stop Feedback

Set Time   1
Metaspace   % Rectified
Harness   % Complete   66

Transfer To Digestive   Transfer To Nerves
Transfer To Circulation   Transfer To Lymph
Transfer To Eyes/Ears   Transfer To Muscles
Transfer To Respiratory   Transfer To Bones

SELECT BIO-SPECIFIC

Nasal Polyps
Sinus Congestion
Sinus Headache
Relieve Pressure

ADD EMPHASIS

Inflammation
Infection
Degeneration
Pain

Click Item To Select View Information Right

ID	Item Name
45	Sinus Headache
46	Sinusitis
47	Sinusitis & immune dys.
48	Sore Throat
49	Strep throat
50	Taste Disorder
51	Throat tumor

Bio-Specific Stress   Anatomical

Sinus headaches are the result of when the ducts connecting the sinuses become swollen. Pressure is then caused in the membrane lining of the nasal passages. These types of headaches can be painful over, behind and under the eyes, extending into the cheeks and upper jaw bone. They can be extremely painful and uncomfortable.

Sinus headaches are often relieved with some type of decongestant. Decongestants are not for everyone, so discuss the options with your family physician. The key is to unclog the congested sinuses to relieve the pressure before the sinuses become infected.

Sinus obstruction can be caused by allergic reactions to things like airborne pollens, dust, animal dander, molds, as well as foods.

2 Min Spec Stim

72

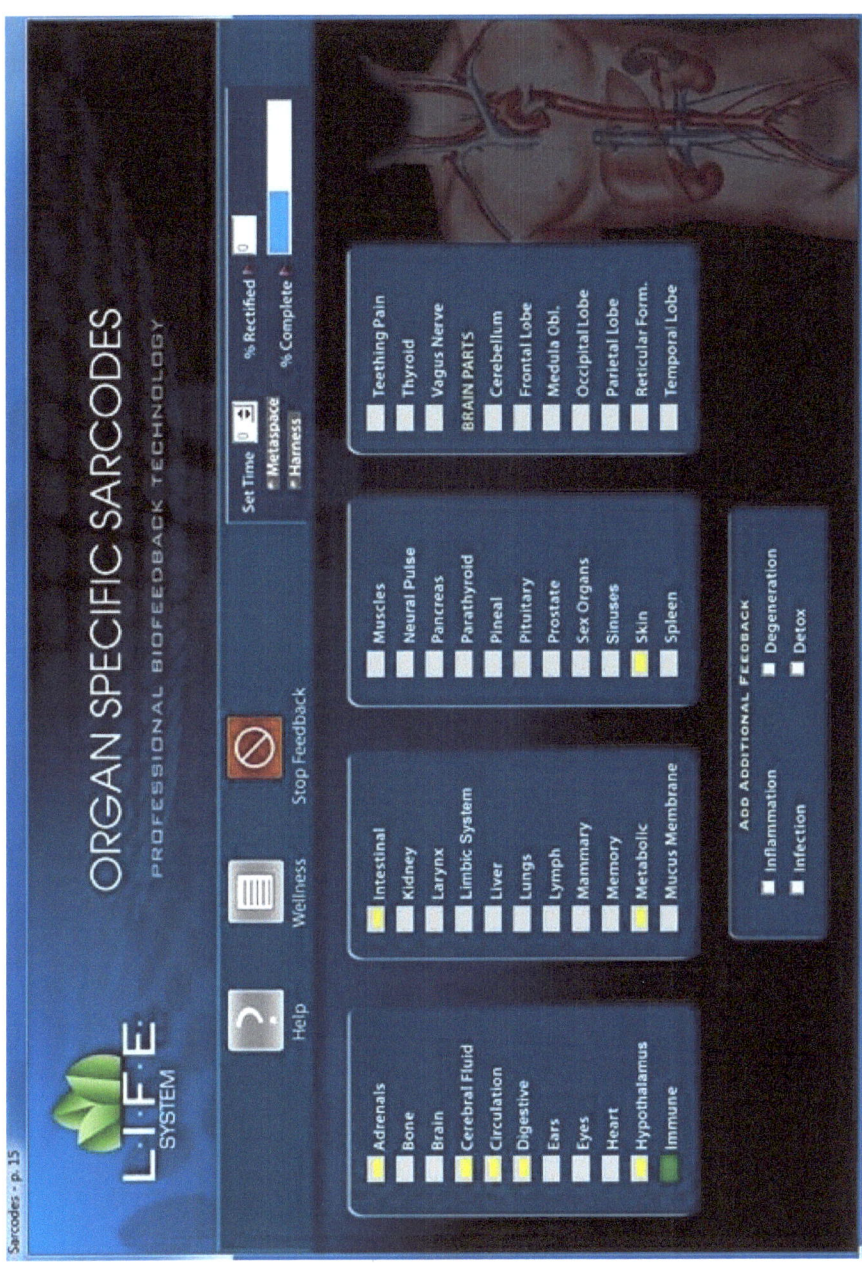

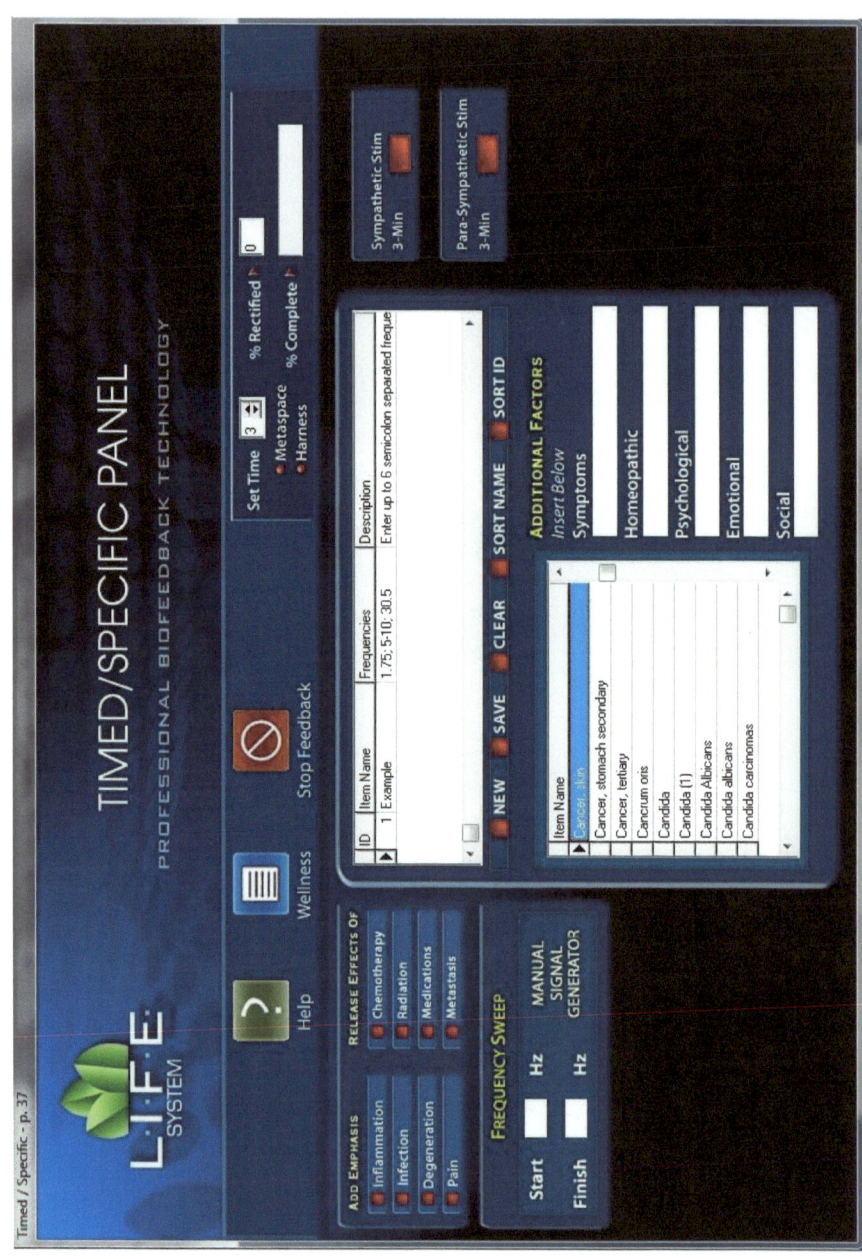

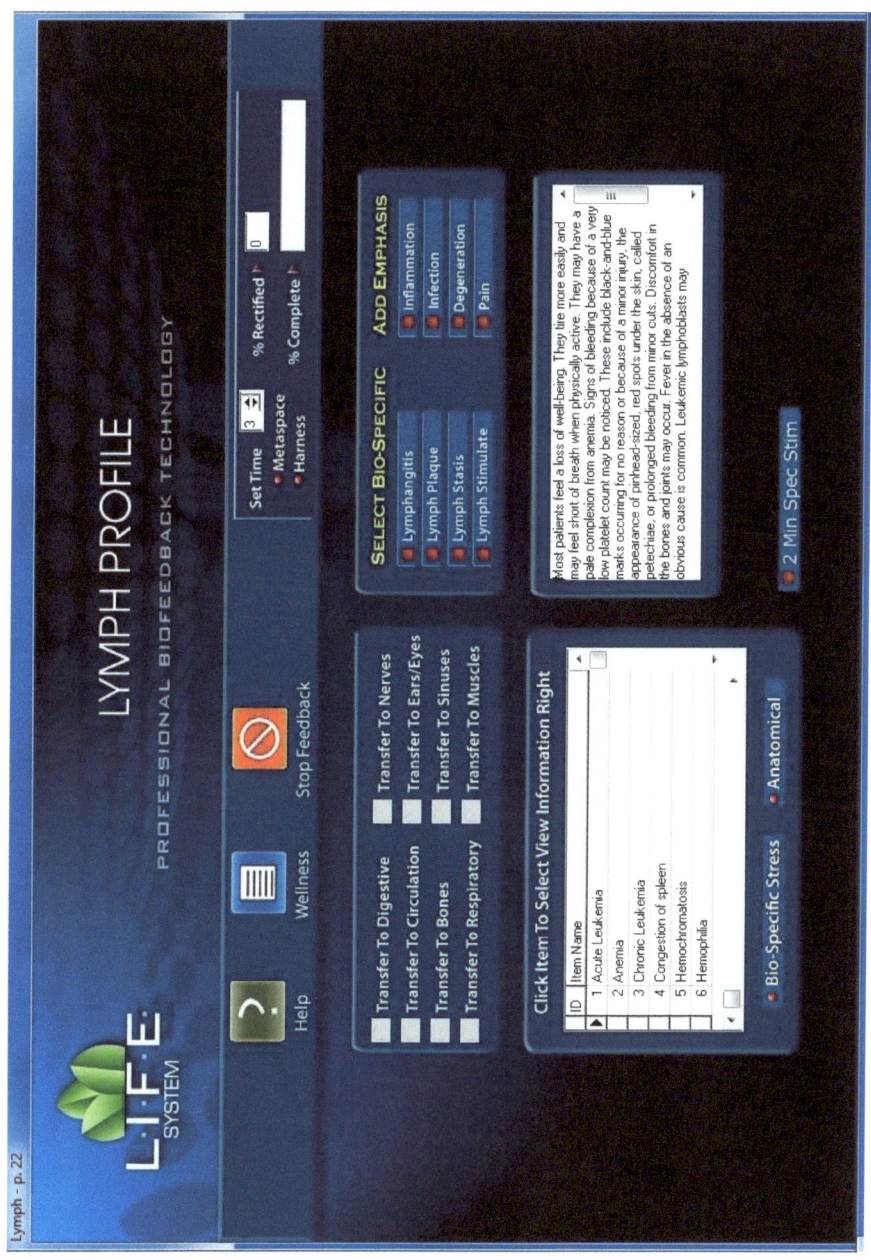

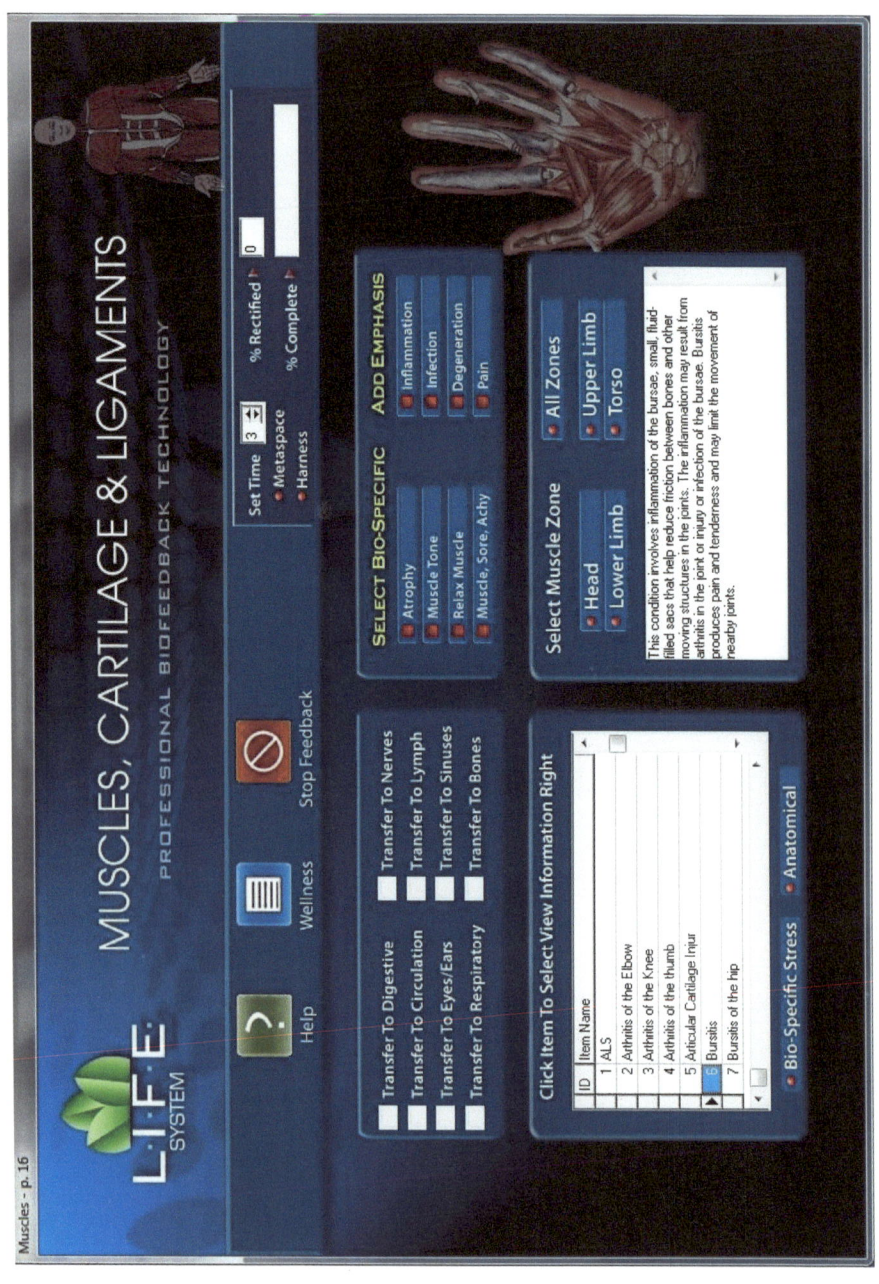

MUSCLES, CARTILAGE & LIGAMENTS

PROFESSIONAL BIOFEEDBACK TECHNOLOGY

L·I·F·E
SYSTEM

Help   Wellness   Stop Feedback

Transfer To Digestive   Transfer To Nerves
Transfer To Circulation   Transfer To Lymph
Transfer To Eyes/Ears   Transfer To Sinuses
Transfer To Respiratory   Transfer To Bones

Click Item To Select View Information Right

ID	Item Name
1	ALS
2	Arthritis of the Elbow
3	Arthritis of the Knee
4	Arthritis of the thumb
5	Articular Cartilage Injur
6	Bursitis
7	Bursitis of the hip

Bio-Specific Stress   Anatomical

Set Time 3
Metaspace
Harness

% Rectified   0
% Complete

SELECT BIO-SPECIFIC
Atrophy
Muscle Tone
Relax Muscle
Muscle, Sore, Achy

ADD EMPHASIS
Inflammation
Infection
Degeneration
Pain

Select Muscle Zone
Head
Lower Limb

All Zones
Upper Limb
Torso

This condition involves inflammation of the bursae, small, fluid-filled sacs that help reduce friction between bones and other moving structures in the joints. The inflammation may result from arthritis in the joint or injury or infection of the bursae. Bursitis produces pain and tenderness and may limit the movement of nearby joints.

www.ingramcontent.com/pod-product-compliance
Lightning Source LLC
Chambersburg PA
CBHW040829180526
45159CB00001B/115